"[A] fascinating book about the unique experience of death and dying within African American culture. . . . By weaving interviews, historical accounts, and personal reflection, Holloway demonstrates how a combination of racial injustice, violence against blacks, and medical neglect has shaped black people's expected transition between this world and the afterlife. . . . [It] may help physicians today understand why some African Americans do not fully trust our present medical system."

—BRIAN C. REED, MD, *Journal of the American Medical Association*

"Karla Holloway writes about a central and little-explored American phenomenon with a wide and patient breadth of knowledge and a startlingly profound personal depth. It feels like a book as durable as a well-shaped stone—as reliable, useful and finally consoling, however hard to bear."

—REYNOLDS PRICE, author of *Ardent Spirits: Leaving Home, Coming Back*

"Beginning with the tragic loss of her son, Karla Holloway poignantly examines how race not only affects the meaning of black lives, but their deaths as well."

—PAULA GIDDINGS, author of *When and Where I Enter: The Impact of Black Women on Race and Sex in America*

"[A] stunning portrait of African American death in the 20th century that includes discussions of the business of funerals and wakes, the ways African Americans die (using a host of statistical analysis), and the place of the black church and funeral ceremonies in African American culture. One of the particularly startling points of *Passed On* is Holloway's inclusion of her son's death in her prologue and his funeral sermon at the end. *Passed On* is a valuable book because it is able to articulate distinct social practices, and ultimately show how death pervades not only African American life, but identity."
—*Virginia Quarterly Review*

"Holloway weaves a seamless and engaging narrative from interviews, historical sources and personal testimony, showing continuity in the black experience of death. . . . Her tales are by turns poignant, horrifying and amusing."
—JOSIE APPLETON, *Times Literary Supplement*

"Punctuated with Holloway's personal stories (including that of her son's death), the book is an elegantly written survey for general readers and cultural historians alike."
—*Publishers Weekly*

"[An] engaging and, at times, heartbreaking, study of death in African American culture . . . [Holloway] demonstrates how cultural and academic criticism can, and should, have a personal effect, both for those who write it and for those who read it. It is a lesson she learned well from W. E. B. Du Bois."
—ERIK BLEDSOE, *ForeWord*

"The threatening possibility of injury, abuse, and premature death stalks black lives in America as the moving *Passed On* poignantly evidences. . . . Holloway's description of how the prison overseer galloped after [her son], shooting him in the back 17 times is chilling and sensitizes the reader to keep at the front of their mind the sorrowful dimension inherent in her topic."
—KAY BOURNE, *Bay State Banner* (Boston)

"Holloway's book is a survivor's tale, itself built on remembrances of survivors. . . . Higher praise is hard to express."
—JOHN SAILLANT, *Chicken Bones: A Journal*

"[T]his powerful, moving, and frequently upsetting book is welcome. It speaks to a deep sorrow in the African American zeitgeist. . . . *Passed On* ventures close to places many folks would rather not go. [Holloway's] courage and empathy are apparent throughout this path-breaking book."
—TIM HASLETT, *Black Renaissance/Renaissance Noire*

"Filled with research on gut-wrenching details of lynchings and sometimes shoddy undertaking practices, and recounting many personal stories, the book is both hard to read and hard to put down."
—LYNDA ZIMMER, *The News-Gazette* (Champaign-Urbana, Illinois)

"*Passed On* is a well-researched and beautifully written book. . . . [A] memorable text that dares to affirm and celebrate black life even in the midst of the conditions of death."
—ALTON B. POLLARD III, *Alabama Review*

"This well-written history of African American funeral practice encompasses history, narrative, and social science. . . . One is grateful for the store of information provided by Holloway's scholarship, amazed at our resilience given the sometimes horrific history Holloway presents, and awed by the strength of soul that allowed her to conceive this work and bring it to term even as she mourned her own son. *Passed On* is a highly recommended read."
—LINDA I. KIRKLAND-HARRIS, *The African American Pulpit*

PRIVATE

·

BODIES,

·

PUBLIC

·

TEXTS

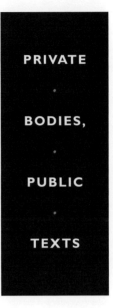

PRIVATE

·

BODIES,

·

PUBLIC

·

TEXTS

Race, Gender, and a Cultural Bioethics

KARLA FC HOLLOWAY

Duke University Press · *Durham and London* · 2011

© 2011 Duke University Press

All rights reserved

Printed in the United States

of America on acid-free paper ∞

Designed by Amy Ruth Buchanan

Typeset in Charis

by Tseng Information Systems, Inc.

Library of Congress Cataloging-

in-Publication Data appear on the

last printed page of this book.

This book is dedicated

to the memory of my sister,

Karen Andrea,

who lived a loving life

of interdisciplinary

intelligence and grace.

She blessed us all.

Stories are lived
before they are told.

—Alasdair MacIntyre,
After Virtue

Contents

Preface

Private Bodies, Public Texts is an interdisciplinary meditation on literature, legal studies, and bioethics that constitutes a theory of cultural ethics. In a Web search for "cultural ethics," the results would include references to "ethics in culture" and "cross-cultural ethics." Cultural ethics is different from these in three very important ways.

First, it is a methodology that insists on cultural complexity as the origin of subjectivity. For bioethics, this means a primary and focused consideration of the habits, patterns, and practices in medicine and law that subsequently constitute the discipline's subjects. In other words, cultural ethics acknowledges that the discursive practices of the field—the complexities of history, institutions, and their texts—produce the field.

Second, cultural ethics acknowledges that ethical inquiry is not empty of social histories, nor does it discount the regulatory heft of institutionalized practices of cultural conduct. This acknowledgment engages the necessarily unwieldy exchange between subject and subjectivity—the discursive subject as text and the narrative idea of personhood. One way this book notices the slippery constitution of subjectivity is in its use of literary texts as methodology.

Its particular attention to narrative as text, the third difference of cultural ethics, displays the ways in which narrative is not a mere abstraction from a disciplinary field onto a body of inquiry. Consider, for example, the consequentialist effects of bioethics' focus on the "patient's story," which has also been a familiar focus of narrative ethics. Cultural ethics, however, interrogates the architectures of knowledge and its forms of production that contribute to the shape of disciplinary knowledge. In other words, the histories of bioethics' interests, including the revelatory focuses within the field's vocabularies, are constitutive structures. Bioethicists' focused abstraction of a "patient's story" actually formulates an interrogative for a theory of cultural ethics.

Harriet Washington's *Medical Apartheid* offers an interesting example of the productive differences excavated within the complex terrain of cultural ethics, where issues of social justice, historical pattern, scientific efficiency, legal standing, and economics contribute to the science and practice of medicine and the interests of a more traditional understanding of bioethics.[1] The integrity of Washington's compelling narrative regarding habits of medical research that have been a consistent feature of U.S. medicine illustrates the focus of a cultural interrogation of history's patterns, and the difference of this focus from traditional practices of bioethics in its collection and review of cases, narratives, and events in medical research with less attention to their intersectionality than to their exemplary stories. Bioethics' subjects are constituted as objectified phenomena of the field—the interests of its Hurstonian "spy-glass."

A cultural ethics follows the critique implicit in Foucault's 2006 lectures at the Collège de France, in which he notes that "the relationship of sovereignty is a relationship in which the subject-element is not so much, and we can even say it is almost never, an individual, an individual body. The relationship of sovereignty applies *not to a somatic singularity but to multiplicities*" (emphasis added).[2] Following these parameters, a cultural ethics does not merely notice the ethical lapse that yields a case narrative about (for example) elderly Jewish nursing home residents whom American researchers injected with live cancer cells in an experiment on immune system response; or minority children and their families from Baltimore who were assigned to public housing known to be infested with dangerous levels of lead, in the Kennedy Krieger Institute studies. The subjects of those cases are not somatic singularities, but multiplicities. A cultural ethics considers what it is about the constitution of those subjects and the patterns and cultures of medicine that make it possible, even predictable, to repeat these kinds of ethical failure. Foucault properly notes that a "somatic singularity is effectively marked with the seal of the sovereignty that accepts it."[3]

Even though this book claims bioethics as its disciplinary location, and to the degree that bioethics is concerned with the body, the sovereignties under interrogation here include the field of bioethics as a body of textual practice. This book's interest in cultural ethics names the sustained practice of Washington's *Medical Apartheid* and places narratives that engage race and gender directly into the substantive issues of bioethics' contemporary interests. It does so with a decided bias regarding the structures of narrative.

The bias of *Private Bodies, Public Texts* lies within its presumption that bioethics' practiced objectification of patients' (and sometimes physicians') stories in its contemporary regard for narrative medicine's "honoring" the stories of illness erases a critical textual feature.[4] The objectification of a patient's story fails to give constitutive weight to the cultural and historical context of that experience. The irony is that these contexts have often been explicitly shaped by the field of medicine. In my judgment, narrative medicine cannot ignore the intersections and histories embedded in the thick cultures within science, medicine, law, and society that have produced the very stories that are of such interest to the field.

The idea of this book is not to merely fill in the histories and cultural milieu that form contemporary narratives of interest to bioethics, but to claim the multiplicities in these otherwise disciplinary narratives. Narrative attention to history and culture cannot fully imagine the rest of the story for events like the Tuskegee syphilis study, or the birth control trials in Puerto Rico, or the gendered dimensions of publicly riveting right-to-die cases. In order to engage this more complicated terrain, this book uses fiction to resist the thin and focused habits of objectification and to suggest instead that a subject's constitution might be considered as complex and elusive, rather than readily available. One is reminded of the ethnographer Zora Neale Hurston's naive question "do you know any stories?" on her first (failed) field trip into the American South. She returned to her Columbia University mentor, Franz Boas, distressed and disheartened by this failed effort. But cultural ethics is not only interested in exemplary stories of ethical practice. Instead it gives prima facie acknowledgment to the cultures that have produced those stories, and—despite the evidence in cases that bioethics excavates for our consideration—cultural ethics excavates and then interrogates the patterns of the field's interest.

In retrospect, I've been at this work a long time—at least since my 1995 *Codes of Conduct: Race, Ethnicity and the Color of Our Character*, and certainly in my books that have explored the cultural history of black death and dying in the United States: my 2002 *Passed On: African American Mourning Stories; A Memorial* and my 2006 examination of the cultures of reading in *BookMarks: Reading in Black and White; A Memoir*.

The four essays that focus the chapters of *Private Bodies, Public Texts* (on reproduction, clinical trials, genomics, and death and dying) seem, and can certainly be approached as, discrete. But in fact they intersect in ways that mirror a theory of cultural bioethics. The cases in medical ethics and law that emerge from these essays involve matters of identity—race and gender, in particular. This was my intent. But it was a surprise to discover that the idea of privacy was a mediating and indeed a coordinating consideration for these chapters—despite their different focuses. It became very important to the organization and composition of this book to understand the consequence to the value of the private when identities like race, age, ability, and gender are visibly evident or nominatively in play. In searching for a way to conduct this important inquiry in bioethics, I turned to literary texts in order to tell the rest of the story.

Narrative ethics is a disciplinary focus in bioethics that uses literature to illustrate matters of ethical concern and to assist listeners in hearing a patient's story in order to develop a more thoughtful perspective on treatment. The idea of story is paramount in narrative ethics, and allocating value to a patient's story is one way of shifting the dynamics of authority that are so vigorously embedded in medicine. My interest in narrative certainly springs from my background in literary studies. But my legal background and experience with medical ethics also contribute to my interest in the cultural construction of narrative. As a scholar rather than a practitioner, I have what I readily acknowledge as the liberty to be less interested in sussing out an expedient and judicious solution, which is the appropriate destination of medical (and legal) ethics. Instead of engaging literary narratives in order to select facets of these stories that we might apply to ethical solutions for medical or legal issues, this book uses narratives to underscore the ways in which culture is a vigorously constructed interplay of identities—illustrative of Foucault's "multiplicities." Cultural bioethics insists on a generative perspective that establishes ethical paradigms as fully entangled in identitarian presumptions.

Finally, a note regarding the consequence of my decision to focus on gender and race. Gender in this book does not mean white women. It means the social constructions of women, or of men. Even though our academic lens has been (inappropriately, in my judgment) primed to see race and gender as discrete categories, the fact is that males and females both have racialized bodies. The importance of Tuskegee in my analyses is that it includes the category of males as well as that of black racialized bodies. Sometimes one facet of identity seems the issue that is provocative. For example, right-to-die cases focus on women who reach the media's attention. But the fact is that it is white women in these high-profile stories who have become icons of the media. There are men who suffer these end-of-life indignities, as well as people of color; but we cannot recall the names and bodies at issue in these cases with as much ease as we can name the white women who have earned national attention. Why not? Because race matters. Notice the similarity of these cases to the plethora of public stories of missing white women and girls that gain extraordinary and sustained media attention. The stories of other missing persons—men and boys, women and girls of color—are absent from the national attention and public focus. Race and gender have a complicated interplay, and this text's consideration of these social categories attends to that interplay.

For cultural ethics, the question is not how does a body's personhood matter? Rather, it is in what ways is the *presumption* of a body's *culturally constructed* personhood relevant to ethical inquiry? And what are the regulatory frames that accompany our interrogations? A critical argument of this book is that these answers reside differently in private

lic spheres. My thinking here is deeply informed by my response
ling of Judith Butler—most specifically the considerations in
is Life where she explains how "the public sphere is constituted
y what cannot be said and what cannot be shown. The limits of
the sayable, the limits of what can appear, circumscribe the domain in
which political speech operates and certain kinds of subjects appear as
viable actors."[5] Butler's "viable actors" are bioethics' vulnerable populations—those whose personhood is attenuated by their corporeal status
under the law or within social constructions. When Butler proposes that
a "grievable death"—one that is both noticeable and sayable in the public sphere—is determined through "normative schemes of intelligibility
[that] establish what will and will not be human, what will be a livable
life, what will be a grievable death,"[6] she references precisely the conundrum that arises when human legibility is determined by a stratified
recognition of personhood. Public discourse proceeds from the versions
of legibility that certain bodies produce.

In conclusion, an important note on the process of the book remains.
It is sprinkled with questions. It is my hope that their rhetorical nature
will encourage additional discussion or thinking and illustrate the multiple locations of critique that might be provoked when we use the idea
of the private to negotiate identity, bioethics, and narrative.

Acknowledgments

I am grateful for the forums that provided the intense intellectual engagement that allowed me to develop the ideas of this book. Among them, the W. E. B. Du Bois Institute at Harvard University was a scholarly haven. Henry Louis Gates's gracious welcome of me into that community came at a critical juncture that allowed my scholarship to reclaim itself from a torrent of local politics that threatened to overwhelm. I thank my Du Bois Institute colleagues for their conversations and coffee, lectures and lunches, and for the way in which they live so brilliantly the life of the mind in that ideal space.

Professor Randy Kennedy at Harvard Law School kindly extended to me a space in his lively and thoughtful class titled Race Relations in the 20th Century, and those interludes, as well as our deeply engaging and delightful conversations, improved significant parts of my thinking with regard to the issues of race in this book. Ellie Nowak, a Harvard undergraduate, met my requests for research and review with good will and an indomitable spirit. I am indebted to her intelligent and careful readings of early drafts as well as her considerable talents, offered without condition and with an intellectual curiosity that inspires. I am grateful as well to Sharon Harley for extending the space of her friendship to the Vineyard retreat.

My colleagues and students at Duke University, especially in the English department; the John Hope Franklin Humanities Institute; African

& African American Studies; the Trent Center for Bioethics, Humanities and the History of Medicine; the Duke Institute on Care at the End of Life; and the Duke University Law School have been consistently supportive, warmly encouraging, and intellectually engaging. I am grateful for their confidence and their kind and courageous collegiality.

There are cohorts of friends and colleagues who deserve special mention here, and I am grateful to them all. The Friday Night Women's Book Club and Wintergreen Writers' Collective remain a source of loving kindness and friendship. My colleagues on the Greenwall Foundation's Bioethics Advisory Board—Baruch Brody, Robert Burt, Christine Cassell, Bernie Lo, and the foundation's director, Bill Stubing—have been rigorous and thoughtful in the formation of our community of bioethics scholars. I am grateful for the engaged and provocative conversations and their own dedicated and inspiring scholarship on some of the very issues that are my focus in this book. *Private Bodies, Public Texts* is indebted, in no small measure, to the sustained and invaluable seminars on bioethics that our meetings and deliberations have created. The DNA, Race and History group—especially the leadership and support of Keith Wailoo, of Rutgers University, and Alondra Nelson, of Columbia University—provided a critical sounding board and a collegial community to share my interests in genomics and race. My election as a Hastings Center Fellow promises an exciting venue for sharing the ideas in this book and learning from a stellar group of bioethicists. I am grateful to the members of the Hastings Center Board for their invitation to join this esteemed company.

Ken Wissoker of Duke University Press was immediately encouraging of this project several years ago when I approached him with the idea of an anthology, and he suggested that I consider instead a monograph on the critical issues that could be framed within a theory of cultural bioethics. I am supremely fortunate that his was a consistent and encouraging voice at the beginning of this project, and especially that he remained as interested and supportive once it became the book he had the foresight and confidence to imagine. Duke University Press is an ideal space for new scholarly directions and is open and encouraging of the ideas and intersections that emerge when this kind of scholarship is nurtured. Ken Wissoker's professionally astute judgment regarding cultural studies was evident in every step of the press's expert and informed approach to the book, including his selection of a critically engaged and intellectually rigorous group of anonymous readers. Their careful attention and detailed commentary made the final manuscript significantly better. Rebecca Fowler and Jeanne Ferris brought a critical and polished professionalism to the final manuscript for which I am absolutely indebted. Their work is evident in the ways the book succeeds; any errors or lacunae are, of course, my own.

Kate Bartlett, Lauren Dame, Ruth Faden, Kerry Haynie, Wendy Harris, Margaret Humphreys, Nancy M. P. King, Wahneema Lubiano, Anne Lyerly, Paula McClain, Richard Payne, H. Jefferson Powell, Charmaine Royal, Maurice Wallace, Harriet Washington, and John Weistart have, in various ways, gone well above whatever is ordinary in professional and collegial support, and I thank each of them for the keen intelligence that they have so generously shared. Susan Reverby is certainly a member of that company, but she is due a very particular thanks. Susan not only shared her own model of scholarly dedication and focus, but she also extended her considerable expertise and rigorous intelligence to me with genuine courtesy. A special thanks remains for me to extend to the colleague whose own brilliantly composed intellectual life remains inspiration and assurance: I am better for the attentive concern and the fierce intelligence of Professor Robyn Wiegman.

And finally, I express my absolute gratitude and devotion to my husband Russell, my daughter Ayana, and her husband Javier Arce. Each selflessly brings mind, heart, and spirit to each of our days. They must know these are tremendous gifts, and how deeply the greatest of these—love—sustains.

PRIVATE

·

BODIES,

·

PUBLIC

·

TEXTS

The Law of the Body

Terri's Law • After Terri Schiavo had been in a persistent vegetative state for nearly fifteen years, her husband, Michael, attempted to end her prolonged dying. A respirator and a feeding tube had kept her breathing and provided her body with sustenance following the respiratory and cardiac arrest that she experienced in her Florida home in 1990. Michael sought to end the artificial life support, a decision he felt his wife would have made for herself had she been competent to do so. After years of fruitless efforts to alter his wife's state, he finally petitioned for removal of the medical devices and, as her legal guardian by marriage, he attached a do not resuscitate order to her medical records. His decision was opposed by her parents, and the court battles that ensued to contest her parents' attempts to halt the removal of the tubes brought publicity to the case. In an extraordinary move for such a private family matter, her parents' efforts were eventually supported by the Florida legislature, which passed "Terri's Law"—legislation that effectively gave Jeb Bush, then the state's governor, authority to intervene in the case.

An appeals court ruled that Terri's Law was unconstitutional. But before that ruling, there was an unprecedented public intervention in what one might have reasonably considered a private family matter. Following the verdict by Florida's Second District Court of Appeals to adhere to her husband's decision to remove the feeding tube—a decision fought by her parents—the U.S. Senate passed legislation that allowed it to enter the family's quarrel, and a bill called the "Palm Sunday Compromise" was introduced in the House of Representatives, requiring that the Florida case be moved from state to federal jurisdiction. Outside of the nursing home where Terri lay dying, Randall Terry, a right-to-life activist, orchestrated noisy public demonstrations to protest Michael Schiavo's efforts.

The legions of protestors outside of the nursing home ensured that Terri's dying would be a public spectacle. Michael's decision to end her life ultimately prevailed, and Terri Schiavo died on March 21, 2005. On her tombstone are two death dates: 1990 and 2005. Too many people know the intimate details of what might have been a private family tragedy.

Henrietta's Haunting · On the day in October 1951 when Henrietta Lacks died of ovarian cancer in Baltimore, Maryland, her husband and children completed the necessary paperwork to release her body from the hospital morgue and sorrowfully began to make the funeral arrangements that would return the body of their wife and mother to her home for burial. The grief-stricken family was fully engaged in the business of her burial. They had no idea that on that very evening, Dr. George Gey, a tissue culture researcher at Johns Hopkins University, where she had been a patient and had died, had convened a press conference. Clutching a test tube that contained cells from her tumor, cells that his laboratory had collected months earlier, he announced that a new era of medical research had begun—one that, someday, could produce a cure for cancer. The family knew nothing of Gey's television appearance, nor had they any idea that cells had been harvested from Henrietta's tumor.[1]

Some twenty-five years later, Barbara Lacks, the wife of one of Henrietta's sons, was invited to a friend's home. The friend had also invited her sister and brother-in-law to dinner. The brother-in-law was a scientist from Washington, and after introductions and some conversation, he reportedly turned to Barbara and said: "Your name sounds so familiar . . . I think I know what it is . . . I've been working with some cells in my lab; they're from a woman called Henrietta Lacks. Are you related?" "That's my mother-in-law," Barbara whispered, shaking her head, "She's been dead almost twenty-five years, what do you mean you're working with her cells?"[2]

Even before Henrietta Lacks succumbed to the ovarian cancer that had spread throughout her body, the cells from the tissue culture taken from her tumor were already exhibiting an extraordinary vitality. In the first quarter-century after her death, her cell line had become legendary in research labs around the world. The sociobiologist Hannah Landecker perceptively explains the vitality of the cell line (known as HeLa) developed from Henrietta Lacks's tumor. Landecker writes: "HeLa continues to be used, explained, exploited and narrated in the scientific and popular press, as well as through film and television, making it one of the most *storied* biological entities of the twentieth century" (emphasis added).[3] Landecker's acute understanding of the unusual circulation of this event is reflected in her vocabulary: she notes "the personification of the cell line in the image of the woman from whose body it was extracted." That night over a dinner table, two worlds collided. One was private and involved a family who still mourned the death of their mother. The other was public and concerned a scientific community that had been using her tissue cultures to grow cell lines for a wide variety of medical research. Until that moment and the later publicity that came to be attached to Henrietta Lacks, the family had borne their loss privately, and medical research had profited from the vitality of a cell line that became immortal (another personification) and the product of Microbiological Associates, Inc., the biological supply company that made the cells available for commercial use.

The robust utility of the tissue sample taken from Henrietta Lacks was indeed extraordinary. Like no other human cellular material before it, the cervical cancer cells that came from Henrietta Lacks had a remarkable vitality. Before the recovery and use of her tissue samples, there were no immortal human cancer cell lines—that is, there were no human cells that did not eventually experience cell death, or apoptosis. Mrs. Lacks's cells did not die. The science reporter Michael Gold describes what happened to the cells from her tumor:

At some point, the cells in each little island of tumor began to quiver and dance . . . and multiply. Where there had been one, there were now two. Where there had been two, now four, now sixteen, now thirty-two. In a few days, the signs of growth were visible: around each cube [of extracted tissue] a translucent band of new cells was taking shape . . . Every other human cell line in the Gey lab had faltered. Yet as the months passed, the HeLa cells showed no such vulnerability. They just kept growing, doubling their number every twenty-four hours . . . the tumor cells were growing ten to twenty times faster than the normal cervical tissue taken from Henrietta Lacks.[4]

George Gey, the Hopkins scientist who was head of the tissue culture lab, had given instructions that all cultures taken from cancer patients should be presented to his lab for analysis. An article in the *Johns Hopkins Magazine* described the sample taken from Henrietta Lacks: "They multiplied like nothing anyone had seen. They latched to the sides of test tubes, consumed the medium around them, and within days, the thin film of cells grew thicker and thicker."[5] The discovery was extraordinary and changed the field of medical research. But the same aggressive growth that appeared in the laboratory attacked Henrietta Lacks. Her cancer spread to almost every organ of her body, and nine months after she was diagnosed, she died. Until that coincidental dinner table conversation some twenty-five years later, her family had no knowledge that Henrietta's biological material had entered the public domain and had become the stuff of medical legend.[6] However, many thousands of medical researchers knew of the HeLa cell line's extraordinary ability to multiply. And some, like the dinner table guest, knew Henrietta Lacks's name.

George Gey's interest in keeping that name private had been overridden by Roland Berg, director of scientific information for the National Foundation for Infantile Paralysis, who had professed his expertise in working with the public with this "type of material" and had told Gey that "you do not engage the attention of the reader unless your story has basic human interest elements."[7]

The Washington scientist invited to dinner with Henrietta Lacks's daughter-in-law knew the name of the source of the cell line that made his research possible because there had been a decided effort and specific intent to attach narrative elements to this unusual medical story, despite the fact that the Lacks family was never told that her cells were available to medical researchers. Landecker perceptively weaves the critically constructed narrative into the scientific utility of the cells:

> The widespread presence of the cells in laboratories was equated with the ongoing, if distributed, presence of the woman's life essence. In this period, the personification of the HeLa cells in the figure of Henrietta Lacks was a beneficent one, a story of unfortunate death turned to the benefit of mankind in conquering polio. The cells were understood to be a piece of Henrietta Lacks that went on growing and dividing, encased in a test tube instead of a body . . . Their concomitant personification was in the form of an angelic figure, an immortalized young Baltimore housewife, thrust into a kind of eternal life of which such a woman would never dream.[8]

It was also an "eternal life" that had not been officially revealed to her heirs and descendants. The rest of the text of this narrative is invested with the consequential remnants of her racialized identity. Her "angelic" persona fell away when the cell line was somehow contaminated, likely in one of the many laboratories that circulated the material. Following this new reference for the HeLa line—that it was not a pure sample but a contaminated one—that same personification that attached to her altruistic (albeit unknowing) gift of her body's most intimate material, Lacks's own identity—understood fully as a black woman—was rendered vulnerable to the social stereotypes habitually attached to race and sex. The vocabulary that described the HeLa cell line as "vigorous," "aggressive," and "difficult to control" was not detached from the body that produced them. Stereotypes of black women have historically used that kind of imagery.[9] The disciplined image of Mrs. Lacks that appears with the discussion of HeLa cells has incorporated the very stereotypes— of authoritative power and aggressive dominion—that black women of her era struggled against.

Among the most intimate, most extraordinarily private moments of our lives are those that involve contraception and birth, medical interventions that through experimental or standard care seek to alter the quality of our lives, the event and occasion of our dying, and when we learn more about our biological lives—the remarkably personalized data that is available through genomics and discoveries of the unique information about ourselves that is attached to our DNA. Each of these areas—broadly engaged in this book's four chapters, which focus on reproduction, genomics, clinical trials, and death and dying—has the potential to have an inordinate effect on the ways in which we manage our daily lives. These are experiences that seem universal. But they are decidedly particular as well. Because of the unique cultural and social histories attached to specific populations in the United States, each of these areas has an impact on women and on minorities that inevitably questions our presumptions regarding individual autonomy. At their root, matters of identity are attached to the cultural ideologies regarding a person's fundamental right to privacy.

Private Personhood • In the United States, privacy has a value that is intimately attached to the history of our laws, as well as to the social evolution of our attitudes regarding difference. Gender and race have particular (arguably, peculiar) legal histories in the United States that make the idea of privacy read differently for different bodies. Perhaps as a consequence, or merely in concert with the evolution of differential treatment in the law, our social judgments and cultural perspectives leak into medical practice as well as into advances in science. Of course we are eager to claim and to want science and medical research to be neutral, to concern themselves with facts rather than the politics of identity. But this book argues that social judgments and social systems are critical dimensions of science and medicine. In fact, as medicine reaches toward genomic science for information that might be applicable to individualized therapies, neutrality becomes an even more complicated terrain. Medicine mixes knowledge gained from science and research and knowledge gained from social interaction with a patient.[10] As human as the right to privacy might seem, it has a public history that absolutely renders it a socially selective privilege.

One way to consider the idea of privacy as it is related to the issues of reproduction, genomics, clinical trials, and death and dying is to understand how each of these issues involves the ethics of identity. There is reasonable debate regarding the freedom we have to select our identities, an argument that engages the concept of liberal personhood that John Stuart Mill would champion. But identity is not an insular matter. It is fully shaped by the social narratives that adhere to certain bodies, without concern for or interest in the individual desire for sameness or difference that an autonomous selfhood would assert. Within this frame, sociality is determined by the strength of the identitarian narrative. The most focused consideration of this book is directed toward what it is about race and gender that goes beyond liberal personhood and that controls how identities, rather than persons, interact within the public sphere.[11]

The argument of *Private Bodies, Public Texts* is that narratives— socializing stories—that are attached to all women and to blacks of both genders have an inordinate control over the potential for private personhood. The public controls of race and gender are so robust that private individuation is rarely an opportunity for those whose identities fall within these two social constructs. My consideration of privacy as the ideal but vexed realm of individual personhood explores the ways in which individuality is either subsumed into this nation's social history or extracted from it. The consequence is the compromise of privacy's privilege. We find clear examples of this loss in the ways in which law adjudicates, and medicine practices, disciplinary and regulatory control. The most intimate aspects of our being and the stories that reveal them give shape and contour to a lens that ultimately reveals the loss that women and blacks in the United States experience, as they are woven into collective social categories that separate them from the privileged privacy inherent in the presumptively white and male ideal of liberal personhood.

This book exposes the capaciousness of this loss within legal and medical cases, from legal theory and bioethics. When the legal scholar

Radhika Rao—in an essay on law, medicine, and ethics—poses a question regarding the location of law that might touch property (a legal realm that once included the bodies of enslaved persons), contract (who might enter into such a legal relationship, and who was excluded), and privacy claims, she affirms the narrowed personhood that situates her argument, asking: "Which body of law should become the law of the body?" Rao recalls the case of the Californian John Moore, whose claim to his spleen was denied in a well-known case that held that persons may not claim remnants of their body once it is separated from them. Concerning *Moore v. Regents of the University of California*, Rao writes that "Moore's description of the wrong done to him is quite revealing: 'My doctors are claiming that my humanity, my genetic essence, is their invention and their property.'"[12]

Rao needed Moore's story, as well as his words, to pose her legal questions. Nevertheless, the legal issues were settled without regard to Moore's claim to the integrity of his body as fully human. Other than in depositions or lower court testimonies, a plaintiff's words are not ordinarily found within the decision of an appeals court. At the appellate level, the legal question reigns, and the voices that represent that question are less important than its reach. But Rao uses the voices to great effect in her essay—because the case law insufficiently mined the layered social and cultural narrative that would expand the story. Its complexity was not sufficiently apparent through the plain facts, the legal questions, or the four corners of the final decision.

Moore has reached near legendary status in law and bioethics and is now arguably an ur-text of medical ethics and privacy law. But one of the reasons for its utility is the story's subtext. At least a part of its seminal distinction is that Moore's body was one a reasonable person—the normative standard of the law—might have presumed did indeed belong to him. His gender and his race (he is a white male) placed him among society's most privileged and outside of the coded social identities that have an embedded vulnerability. However, the issue that made the privilege of a private identity *not* the case in Moore's situation—the state's interest in the advance of medical knowledge—is unquestionably worthy of the sustained attention that this case has received in biomedical ethics and property law. Equally significant is the way in which Moore's unexpected occupancy of a privacy and property claim is a telling acknowledgment that there are some bodies who seem to have this entitlement as a normative protection that extends from their citizenship, and there are other bodies who are not only denied this presumption of privacy, but who cannot reasonably anticipate its protection. These other bodies have names and case histories that, even if they are familiar, have not been read into the literature of medical ethics or into the histories of case law within the context of their embodied politics.

My argument in this book is that these other bodies—women and blacks—are bodies that begin with a compromised relationship to privacy. The essential difference between them and John Moore is that their experiences attach to race and gender in ways that Moore's did not. We do not need to know Moore's race or gender in order to read the case, to understand his claim, or to determine its outcome. In law and bioethics reviews, Moore is an individual who was denied a property claim to his body. But those other bodies that make their appearances in law and medicine as distinct and memorable cases, like Terri Schiavo's, often do so through the veil of gender or race. The social categories they occupy do not disappear in objective analyses. In fact, their very subjectivity disrupts their claims to an individual, liberal personhood.

The experiences of women and black Americans are particularly vulnerable to public unveiling. We cannot appreciate the substance of these intimate violations without the accompanying texts of the social identities that govern them. For example, Terri Schiavo was rigorously gendered throughout the frenzied public attention to her plight. She was persistently defined through her familial relationships (as a wife and a daughter), as if those categories by themselves shaped the lens through which the public might more clearly see the dimensions of her tragedy. Privacy is presumed to be a fundamental right of personhood. Nevertheless, particularly for those who made late appearances into constitutional protection, that legal notice has become an assurance that some corporeal feature is always and already vulnerable to public attention as an identity that stands in the place of private personhood. It is as if the Fourteenth Amendment's assurance of equal protection has come to mean that women and blacks would be noticeable first through the legal identity they constitutionally occupy, and only later, and only perhaps, as private persons. What is an appropriate perspective for this vulnerable personhood? One is to acknowledge the thick narratives that reside within the public and the private.

Literary fictions reveal the deeply textured terrains in which stories (or cases) reside. The complex landscapes from which fictional characters emerge might stand in for the texts of fuller narratives that do not often (or appropriately) make it into case law or case histories. The stories that lie between fiction and fact make public narratives resilient. Although law and medicine are rigorously practical fields not much given to the imaginary, literature's stories can encourage our substantive notice and consideration of the ethics embedded within both disciplines. The extended contexts and considered complexities that help us unveil the ways in which privacy and identity matter regarding our perspectives of some bodies benefit from the texture of fiction. Unlike law and medicine, fiction is free to indulge its complications rather than constrained to rigorous enforcement of boundaries that encourage expeditious resolution.

There is good evidence that some of the most compelling fictions use story lines linked to medicine and law. In popular culture, this is why courtroom and hospital dramas so liberally populate some of television's better-known shows. Students in my undergraduate class called Bioethics and Narrative often notice that an issue we are discussing in class appeared in a television show or a film they recently saw.

In the 1960s, television's early heyday, the stories of doctors Kildare and Marcus Welby captivated viewers' attention. In the latter decades of the twentieth century and well into the first decade of the new century, some of television's most popular dramas have been about medicine and law. Audiences are captivated by the issues, characters, and story lines that often take their texts from real-life events. But literary fictions make possible a more complicated life for the legal subject or the medical body than that normally presented in depositions or medical case histories. This more nuanced consideration of complexity is a benefit, especially in fields that try to resolve an issue with expediency. This book's engagement with literary fiction as supplementary material for the ethics-focused analyses of legal and medical narratives is in part specifically because cases in law and medicine are contextually slender. The professional frames of those fields appropriately encourage stripping the story to the essence that results in a lament like John Moore's, that medicine found his humanity in his body's molecular essence rather than in his personhood. In my judgment, our reasoned consideration of the issues that these narratives present stands in need of the nuance that returns the bodies under discussions to full personhood rather than rendering them as essentialized subjects. Fiction is an appropriate and richly textured source for the fully human.

A Patient or a Body? · A physician's comment to me following a talk I gave to the medical humanities group at the Baylor College of Medicine called "The Body Politic" has lingered long past the moment of that lecture. He explained that his aim in teaching was to encourage his students to see patients as people, rather than the disarticulated "bodies" that constituted the topic of my lecture. Bodies are what we have in pathology labs, he explained, but then he went further: "I want my students to understand their patients as human beings—not just human bodies."

I have thought about his comment a good deal and wondered whether it was my inclination, as a cultural studies scholar, to use the language of "the body" in a way that actually belied the point I was making—that the social and cultural have an unwarranted impact on the bodies that are the focus of our medical judgments and the ethics of care.

Both the process and subject of this book are in part a response to the potential of disciplinary divides to separate the subjects of medicine, law, and ethics that would otherwise, it seems to me, find their coherence in a consideration of the body. Instead of distinguishing the legal subject from the patient, and the physician and lawyer from both of these, I want to integrate these subjects into multiple narrative landscapes that examine a dialogic constitution of identity.[13] The result of my effort is this interdisciplinary discussion and focus for this book, with law, medicine, and ethics in conversation with each other and bounded by the thick frames of cultural and literary studies.

Although the shared goal of medical ethics and legal analysis is to find an executable solution to an immediate claim or event, they do so from locations which are both complex and contradictory. The disciplinary approach to legal or medical queries is to pare down the subject to an actionable space, to reduce the scene or event to the legal question or the medical necessity. Whether we appoint an ethics committee to resolve a medical issue or a jury to settle a legal question, we contain these matters within disciplinary constraints that ensure the production of familiar and usable results. Certainly the efficiencies urged in medicine and law are appropriate and necessary; but efficient problem solving is too often achieved by a blind stripping away of material that is textually rich even though it is determined to be "excess" to the cases. I want to urge that, at the very least, we know the excess that we peel away. The messy and unexpected dimensions of fiction might encourage our deliberate engagement with the intricate dimensions of story.

Although the field of narrative bioethics emerged precisely to engage these matters, its focus on patients, physicians, and medical professionals creates a selective universe of actors that influences the judgments and perceptions that patients and medical professionals bring into the arena of medical care. Even when a patient's narrative appropriately occupies the privileged interrogative space, becoming a close reader of—or a more attentive listener to—a patient's story effectively situates that story as a coherent document from which a reading might yield a similarly coherent ethical judgment.

The narrative interest in this book is less about discovering a coherent story which might yield a usable text for a medical professional to read with close attention. As reasonable and well-intentioned as it is to employ "teachers of literature, novelists, storytellers, and patients who have written about their illnesses . . . to attain rich and accurate interpretations of these stories, and to grasp the plights of patients in all their complexity,"[14] another perspective might suggest that there is an inherent tension between the goal of accuracy and the landscape of complexity. Fiction is made up of complexity. It gains its substance from engaging multiple, even contradictory, meanings. Accuracy—the absolutely appropriate goal of law and medicine—is challenged in the fictive environment, and it is the judgment of this book that this challenge is reasonable precisely because of the facts that compose a fictive imagination. The interest of this book is to shift the direction of narrative bioethics away from the disciplinary boundaries that receive a patient's story. Imagine, for example, the common scenario at the doctor's office: "Are you in any pain today? What is the level—from 1 to 10—of your pain?" The questions do not allow for the complex of heartache, the pain of one's spirit. What number might one assign to that?

This book suggests that fiction's sometimes incoherent, messy solutions (if there are solutions at all) and its general tolerance for complexity constitute a narrative that actually fits the rest of the text that a medical professional, no matter how patient a listener or how close a reader, will not be likely to hear from a patient—especially as the questions asked are so strictly regimented. So instead of assigning relative weights to stories told by doctors, nurses, and patients, this book's approach is to look outside of those boundaries for a form of narrative that creates its full and complex stories from the very dilemmas that are capsules in patient care.[15] Additionally, the book interrogates the histories in medicine and law, the cultural texts, that contribute to the stories that narrative bioethics would assign to the patient.

On Privacy, Identity, and Ethics • How does a legal notion of privacy find its way into a cultural narrative? How can privacy articulate a relationship to identity? In bioethics, the traditional engagement with ethics descends from establishing relationships to overarching moral principles (justice, autonomy, beneficence, and nonmaleficence) that moderate and negotiate the solutions that ethical crises demand. These principles encourage our review of ethical quandaries by linking them to the conflicts that might be occasioned in particular circumstances. For example, when the wishes of a patient express the patient's desire for more aggressive care but conflict with a physician's judgment of the futility of further medical intervention, which ethical principles are proffered as the forum for resolution of the dispute? Who is the legal parent—the woman who gestates or the woman who produces the egg? Does race matter? If there is a difference between the race of the zygote and that of the gestational woman, does race matter? Should a woman use selective reduction to choose an embryo that might develop into a tissue match for a child with a terminal illness, who might be saved by the birth of a sibling who could be a donor? Each of these questions takes a private event of the body—illness, pregnancy, or death—and renders it public. The privacy ordinarily anticipated and earned by the intimacy of the event vanishes as certain questions emerge. When there is a public rehearsal of issues, what is the consequence for the bioethical principle of autonomy and the legal right to privacy? What association exists between autonomy and privacy?

These questions involve medical ethics and legal precedents. Medicine and law have designed protocols and doctrinal analyses to regulate the ways in which a solution might be shaped for the problem they represent. Many of these solutions seem finally unsatisfactory to me for two reasons. First, there are cultural questions that can attach to these matters—those that negotiate between privacy and identity—and that are entangled in the solutions. Second, the solutions look outward, toward an objectified subject, rather than inward, at the subjective construction of the discipline. When we utilize the focused perspectives of law or medicine to resolve the dilemmas they represent, matters of culture or identity are either so overregulated that they are stripped of sense, or they disappear into a specific protocol of analytical inquiry.[16] But the textured narratives that are embedded within seem to give both agency and authority to the bodies (disciplinary and corporeal) that center each inquiry. What social judgments about personhood are embedded in the recitation of these stories? How does disciplinary genesis matter when we consider liberal personhood?

Identity matters when private personhood is made public. In a public sphere, where gender or race reign through the force of social construct, historical pattern, and even constitutional authority, social narratives are shaped within the nation's body politic. It is my argument that there are some bodies that will and can ordinarily disappear into the normative, that are not vulnerable to the socialized identity scripts that ensnare public narratives. White male heterosexuals are the unspecified norm against which alternative bodies find themselves publicly visible.

Spectacularity, a hyperpublic notice, exists in direct relationship to ethnicity and gender. In the United States, this has traditionally meant that blacks and women find themselves noticeable in public ways that scan and sculpt perspectives regarding their private personhood. In this national script, the bodies of women and blacks are always and already public.[17]

Writing about the legal doctrine of privacy, the legal theorist Jed Rubenfeld argues that personhood "has so invaded privacy doctrine that it now regularly is seen either as the value underlying the right or as a synonym for the right itself."[18] This invasion creates a conundrum for Rubenfeld, whose essay "The Right of Privacy" considers the central place of sexuality in privacy cases. The social specularity attached to women and blacks explains the focus. Rubenfeld recalls in his essay the provocative notion of an "inviolable personality" and considers it as a flawed but nonetheless cognizable notion of personhood within privacy doctrine.[19] He defines personhood, the center of privacy claims, as "whatever it is that makes you *the* person you are, as opposed to whatever it is that makes you *a* person—a human being." For Rubenfeld, "*the* person" is one who operates in a social context and in the public domain. "*A* person" is the one who is inviolable—simply human. How do *the* private (social) person's acts become not merely human, but vulnerable to public notice? The link between privacy case law and an "individual's personal identity" may or may not interfere with a "personhood thesis." Rubenfeld identifies a riveting result that derives from notice: "the great peculiarity of the privacy cases is their predominant, though not exclusive, focus on sexuality . . . the network of decisions and conduct relating to the conditions under which sex is permissible, the social institutions surrounding sexual relationships, and the procreative consequences of sex."[20]

Legal interest in privacy and *the* body depend on an intimate, gendered, sexual specularity. Locating the legal consideration of personhood within the law's notice of sexuality indicates that a person's private self might be considered an act (rather than a facet) of identity. This reasoning certainly explains the rulings on sodomy cases such as *Bowers v. Hardwick* and *Lawrence v. Texas*.[21] In other words, the law reaches private identity by making private acts public. The issue that makes privacy an act does not depend on the claim to an intimate and ultimately private identity. Instead it rests upon a public expression of that private identity. When Samuel Warren and Louis Brandeis worried in an 1890 essay that what is "whispered in the closets shall be proclaimed from the house-tops," their concern was that the domestic shelter that protected private identities and private acts was vulnerable to public gossip.[22] What acts of identity might these be? Well, what acts of identity, despite their presumptive privacy, are most vulnerable to notice? If they are, as Rubenfeld claims, acts of sexuality, how do we understand the link between sexuality and the ways in which women become the public expression of legal notice? Is identity an act, or some body? We find the answer when we notice which bodies are dislocated from normative gendered and heterosexual privilege.[23]

Rubenfeld is correct to locate the origin of privacy claims in case law that regards (a word that bespeaks the public) expressive sexuality. Although a sense of one's self will certainly develop within the deeply personal and arguably intimate familial context, the making of a person is a complex enterprise. The success of the choices and personalities involved will depend on the manner in which they can be negotiated outside of the private. When I was a youngster, a familiar retort in play-ground battles—as well as from some adults who disapproved of certain conduct—was to "act your age, not your color!"[24] My sisters, playmates, and I took this admonition as a form of rebuke that we were not only being immature, but also acting in a way that made public a noticeably unflattering racial stereotype that attached skin color to conduct. However, there was a positive public claim as well. When we excitedly called friends and family to tell them there was a "black person on TV," it was an acclamation that assured us that in the widest gaze possible (at that moment, television) there was also an acceptable way to be publicly colored.

But there were ethical perils that accompanied public notice—the kind that prompts sometimes voiced, sometimes silent pleas that "I hope it wasn't a black person!" when black Americans hear about a criminal act, perhaps on the radio or in the newspaper. In other words, one could ostensibly win with being publicly colored, but it was also a risk to achieve public notice. Race mattered. For identities with racial or gendered descriptors, the inherent contradiction is that each is as deeply invested in the security implicit in private selfhood as it is in a public sociality. The irony is that the public can supersede and even displace the private.

ETHICS AND AUTONOMY

In *The Ethics of Identity*, the philosopher Kwame Anthony Appiah explains that identity has its own demands, especially in the ways that "our selves are embedded in social forms."[25] Appiah notes that this consequential (public) pluralism—the social forms of self-expression—can challenge "ethical individualism." His argument is a critical notice of private and public selfhood. The ethical individualism enacted in social forms is decidedly public. Is it possible then, that privacy, identity, and ethics might find a shared location? The conjunctive association (ethics and identity) rather than the modified association evident in the title *The Ethics of Identity* is an important syntactic construction that proffers an alliance between ethics and identity. The parallel structure joins these two together and satisfies my interest in linking them to the formations of bioethics' principles. This book's interest in identity begins with its critical association with autonomy—often stated as the first of the four principles that guide traditional bioethics.

Consider autonomy's etymology. It comes from the Greek *autos* (self) and *nomos* (rule). Recalling this etymology explains the importance of a focus on the identitarian (self) nature of authority. Authority, identity, and autonomy are all critical anchors to the discussion in this book. Authority stems from the Latin *auctoritas*—power that is legitimate. An associative argument for a synergistic relationship between autonomy, authority, and individualism encourages a consideration of these as relational terms that see individual liberty and agency as the authoritative (legitimate) construction of the self. Liberty and agency lie at the root of private personhood.[26]

I am a black woman. The plural identities that I claim lie not only in my authority to do so, a private authority that adheres to a selfhood. Because of the evident visibility of the two particular categories my body occupies—gender and race—I actually have little social choice in the matter. My private identities are always and already public.[27]

When value and identity are publicly assigned and associated, it is very often because gender and race are at issue. When identity exceeds the private (that is, when we notice women and blacks essentially because they are not male and white), our notice and the visibility of these categories become a matter of ethical focus.[28] Instead of individual conduct being the initial value of difference, identity produces differential treatment before anything whatsoever is known about individual character. This is especially the case in legal and medical ethics, when the events that are so publicly rehearsed, like the Schiavo case or the utility of Henrietta Lacks's cellular matter, happen in part because the narrative scripts attached to women and blacks become public narratives that very nearly dismiss the private.

Recall the narratives that opened this discussion. Of the "right to die" cases, Terri Schiavo's extraordinarily public and riveting narrative depended on her fitting into the stereotypical categories most often associated with women. She was portrayed as a daughter and a wife in the many retellings of her story. Her tragic situation incorporated all of the historic versions of female helplessness that social histories rehearse. Quite literally, Schiavo could not speak, think, or act on her own behalf. Although these are extreme versions of bias, she fit neatly into those extremes as well as the narratives that we have traditionally attached to the female gender.

Consider, for example, which among the memorable right to die cases are about men. Nancy Cruzan, Terri Schiavo, Elizabeth Bouvia, and Karen Ann Quinlan—the most memorable names associated with these cases are all female. It is certainly true that men have faced the same medical dilemma. But it is the stories of women that make it from the private to public consumption. In the Schiavo case, among those who testified that they knew what Ms. Schiavo would have wanted was her sister-in-law. William Levesque covered her testimony for the *St. Petersburg Times*:

Joan and Terri Schiavo had become close friends in the mid 1980s. Joan Schiavo said she told her sister-in-law about a friend who was forced to end life support to an infant after health problems. Terri Schiavo told her that she would have done the same thing for the baby if its life could not otherwise be saved, Joan Schiavo testified. Joan Schiavo also heard other comments after she and Mrs. Schiavo saw a movie about someone who had an accident and was in a coma. "We had stated that if that ever happened to one of us, in our lifetime, we would not want to go through that. That we would want it stated in our will we would want the tubes and everything taken out. She did not like the movie. Just the whole aspect of family and friends having to come and see their son or friend like that, she thought it was horrible."[29]

Neither Terri Schiavo's own voice nor that of her sister-in-law mattered enough to make state or national legislators honor her wish. The legal spectacle that attached to Schiavo's life was relentlessly gendered in the ways that social context has delivered more authority to men's voices than to women's. The collapse of Schiavo's private identity, nearly obscured in the media circus that surrounded the event of her dying, is a reasonable location for ethical review. The ethics of this matter cannot dismiss the gendered politics in the public space her body came to occupy.

The four chapters of *Private Bodies, Public Texts* encourage our notice of the ways in which race and gender attach to cases in bioethics and law. Recall the case of Henrietta Lacks's tissue culture and cell line. Her family was not informed of the medical discovery associated with her tissue. Why not? Even when medical representatives came to her home to take blood and tissue samples from surviving family members, they misrepresented the purpose of these invasions. What ethical principles were abandoned in these encounters? Did it matter that the family was African American? Does Lacks's case follow any patterns in the medical history of the United States? In other words, is what happened to her predictable?

The pages that follow explore ways in which identity makes particular bodies hypervisible in medical ethics and jurisprudence. Privacy is a privilege that legal and medical interest in identity obscures. The very occasions that we would want to claim as insular, inviolate, and ultimately private are actually—because of the social histories of law and the practices of medicine and research—the most vulnerable, exposed, and critically public. Although a private identity seems a fundamental privilege of personhood, for some it is a fractured privilege. Candice Jenkins, a literary theorist, writes of the paradox of intimacy, noting that "the vulnerability that African Americans have been subject to . . . is the vulnerability of racism . . . bodies too readily exposed."[30]

A critical distinction lies in what Rubenfeld explains as the juxtaposition of *a* (human) person's claim to self-identity and *the* (social) person's acknowledgment of the interior (private) and exterior (public) locations of self. Liberty cannot be a claim of individuality when individual identity is filtered through our associations or assignments to identity categories. Similarly, mirroring the way that an individual cannot liberate herself from the communitarian claims of social personhood, social, political, and legal citizenships have assigned a differential ethical value to particular kinds of citizens at different moments in our history.

This contradiction is engaged in bioethics' considerations of autonomy and the principles that follow it: nonmaleficence, beneficence, and justice. Although it may be easiest to notice or to predict privacy's stake in autonomy, it is also the case that the other principles of traditional bioethics have a substantive relationship to privacy. Whether it is in the medical considerations of harm evident in nonmaleficence and beneficence, or in the legal and ethical notice of justice, in each of these matters (or with regard to each of these principles) the dichotomy of private and public is salient.[31]

With regard to jurisprudence, the history of U.S. constitutionalism has determined that identity absolutely matters to legal process and legal result. In chapter three, I indicate the ways in which rights, as written into constitutional protections, guarantee that identity will be a consistent feature of determining the existence of a legal claim and the manner of a legal solution. Although it would seem that in a democracy, the law should be neutral on its face, our history of jurisprudence has prevented this from being the case. The Civil Rights Act of 1964 and the equal protection clause of the Fourteenth Amendment are primary instruments for claiming that identity matters. In addition, the courts have established standards of judicial review: strict scrutiny for invidious racial discrimination, intermediate scrutiny for cases where gender matters, and rational basis review for cases that do not involve "immutable" identities. However cases are finally decided, and without regard to the judgments we might make regarding the application of the law or our own opinions of the ethical value of the determinations, the structures of legal review are entrenched enough so that for the law, identity is a public, rather than a private, claim.

Chapter 1 of this book, "Bloodchild," considers issues of reproduction, race, and privacy. It opens with a sociohistorical review of how identity has come to matter in the United States and serves as a background to the chapters that follow. In this first chapter, women are certainly the gendered focus. But race is intimately connected to the cultural histories of reproduction in the United States, and for this reason the chapter interrogates gender within and alongside racial identities. What happens differently to white women and minorities in U.S. medicine? Why is poverty a category that can place white women and blacks in a shared vulnerability?

The literary texts that assist the chapter's discussion are an admittedly odd pairing. One is from the twentieth century—a science fantasy story by Octavia Butler. This genre places historical context outside of the frame of analysis because the characters in this story about reproduction (from which the chapter title is taken) are literally alien. The challenge of reading the issues that emerge from legal and medical frames of reproduction into an alien landscape is of no small consequence. But the (literal) alienation of the story brings the biases or presumptions we might have about women or race into focus. How do our presumptions translate into an interpretation of the issue of reproduction if the terrain is imaginary? This consideration renders our presumptions fairly stark in appearance and finally helpful in terms of our notice of difference. But because Butler's story is indeed a stretch, even for fiction, the chapter also offers another fiction—a very short story by the American writer

Kate Chopin, written in 1909. "Désirée's Baby" is a story of paternity—even though the title suggests otherwise. What does the shift in perspective reveal about how we read matters regarding reproduction? And in this story, which has a very visible racial aspect, what happens when our presumptions about race enter a narrative that originally seems to be about reproduction?

Chapter 2 focuses on genomics and is titled "Cartographies of Desire." It follows the chapter on reproduction not only because those issues of biology's minutiae that become public recall the identity of "Désirée's Baby" but also because the ethical issues in genomic medicine have legal consequences. These consequences have been intimately associated with race and with gender. Our understandings of the emerging science of genomics significantly correspond with the social, and with privacy. The fiction that accompanies this telling is also from the twentieth century. However, as with Butler's story, the science in Chopin's is fantastic and futuristic, despite the author's opening claim that locates the story in our "near past." Kazuo Ishiguro's *Never Let Me Go*—a 2005 novel whose startling reality is revealed in this book—gives genomic medicine's potential a landscape that we might readily imagine. The familiar-foreign dichotomy that Ishiguro uses to great effect encourages those interested in bioethics to consider the fate of our ideas about autonomy and justice when medicine and law regulate the social and when the privilege of privacy also means that the state might decide to keep some things secret.

Chapter 3—"Who's Got the Body?"—focuses on clinical trials and research ethics. Perhaps more than any other chapter in this book (although the anecdote is not infrequently recalled), it engages the physician's question to me about bodies and patients, told earlier in this introduction. What are the consequences when clinical trials get reliable data from aggregate subjects rather than individuals? This chapter discusses bioethics' evolution of the idea of "vulnerable subjects"—a term that actually points to the social inequities and judgments that relegate some people to a category of medicine that makes harm more rather than less likely. The conundrum of this chapter is that the focus on the vulnerable becomes a public matter—these are persons whose privacy might mean that we do not notice the ways in which a clinical trial might take advantage of particular identitarian categories.

Bioethics most consistently uses the Tuskegee syphilis study to teach the consequences of ethical oversight (or the lack thereof), but this chapter questions how and why that study became the ur-text for abuse in clinical trials, to the silencing or sublimation of other, equally egregious ethical violations. In its suggestion that the public narrative of sexuality, race, and gender is rehearsed each time that Tuskegee and syphilis are mentioned in the same sentence, the chapter challenges bioethics to consider the cultural reasons why other stories of clinical abuse have disappeared in favor of Tuskegee's texts.

Finally, chapter 4 on death and dying, takes its title "Immortality in Cultures" from a line in Margaret Edson's provocative and elegant drama, *Wit*. Edson's work serves as the literary center of this chapter's analysis on death and dying and bioethics' interest in these narratives. In chapter three, I recall to the discussion the thinking of Owen Barfield, an English philosopher, linguist, and barrister, regarding the differences between a speaker's meaning and text. Barfield's argument in *Speaker's Meaning* is that text is expressively contractive—it reduces meaning in order to communicate intent.[32] It is essentially different from a speaker's meaning, which is expansive with regard to the deep structures of meaning (and experience, socialization, and so forth) that come into play when we hear or use language. The staged performance of Margaret Edson's drama might be both a speaker's meaning as well as a text that a reader engages, a contractive language—words that have been selected for a specific and narrow intent. Of course, literature itself problematizes Barfield's idea here (and what do we do with poetry or spoken texts?). For the chapter on death and dying, that intersectional problem of speaker and text becomes an inquiry—focused on bioethics—into the event and interpretation of the dying during the moment of Hurricane Katrina. A short story by the Harlem Renaissance author Arna Bontemps, "A Summer Tragedy," gives further texture to this chapter.

Although this book consistently regards the dying (within the chapter on clinical trials and even with the immortal cultures of Henrietta

Lacks's cell lines), the play *Wit*, about a death of an English professor for whom words mattered deeply, seemed the most appropriate vehicle to engage the troubled matters of those who died during and after the hurricane named Katrina.

It also seemed a most appropriate conclusion to this study by an English professor who has written on death and dying in a previous study,[33] who has thought deeply herself about the ends of days, and for whom words—with all their intrigue, intellect, intent, and indeed wit— continue to matter. And for the victims of Katrina, they deserved this moment to incorporate this text's final words.

ONE

Bloodchild

This chapter explores the intersections of gender, race, and ethics in contemporary issues in reproduction, and it outlines issues in U.S. history that have rendered women's bodies available for a certain kind of public scrutiny. The nation's
early connection between citizenship and identity contextualizes the evolution
of state interest in intimate matters of sexuality. The histories of scrutiny and
the ethical questions that attach to women and race suggest that contemporary ethical issues in reproductive medicine are not tied to the technologies of
modern birth. Instead, the issues are apparent in the relationship that women's
public and private lives have to their citizenship and the vigorous circulation of
women's bodies in public, legal, and medical discourse. The history of this identitarian relationship, evident in our country's founding cultures, offers an interpretive frame for medical and legal issues in privacy, ethics, and reproduction.
Privacy connects the issues of race and gender from the earliest eras of U.S. history to the contemporary moment.

• • •

Although death was a constant threat to American colonists in the seven-
teenth century, birth was their vital promise. Children who survived the
rugged conditions of the early settlements would not only ensure a future
for New England colonies, but they would develop and sustain the ideals
and principles that led to the nation's founding. The early nation's interest in the fertility of its citizens was intimately attached to the religious
fervor of the English colonists. For Puritans, "be fruitful and multiply"

was a biblical dictum, and "fruitfulness itself conferred status." Pregnancies were viewed as "a contribution . . . to the common task."[1]

A viable nation meant the deliberate and intentional production of (and discernment between) its first citizens. The colonists were not only concerned about their immediate survival. Because the first settlements were seen as religious and political evidence of a particular set of principles, their physical survival was attached to the implementation of those principles. The polity of the nation was substantively embedded in its domestic vision.

The ideals of the new nation followed its expansion across the continent. Early America was necessarily public. Survival depended on everyday commerce and contact between settlers. However, a consequence of the country's growing security and independence was that family life became increasingly insular. Cities displaced communal colonial landscapes, and family homes—once they were removed from the interdependencies of colonial villages—evolved into "a separate place of work, leaving the family domain a private retreat [and] family life as the training ground for citizenship."[2]

One aspect of the loss of interdependency was the consequent escalation of slavery. In terms of reproduction and labor, the bodies of slave women were as vital to the South as white women's had been to the survival of the colonies. Because reliably available populations of enslaved Africans were essential to the plantation economy of the South, manipulating the reproductive capacities of slave women became an economic issue that trumped slavery's ethical problem.[3] The expansion of the population was related to geographical expansion and mirrored associated developments of the nation's legal and social systems. Discoveries in medicine were similarly patterned, focusing on the successful growth and stability of the nation.

The connections between reproductive science and medicine, public policies, and ethics evidence the ways in which these fields are shaped within a national frame and are aligned with the social. Interest in the most intimate and gendered matters of the private body—specifically sexual reproduction—quickly became a matter for national and legal notice. From its founding, the nation had a consuming interest in women's biology. Whether it was the necessary fertility of enslaved black women or white women colonists, women's reproductive potential and the national interest in sustaining and increasing its population rendered women's bodies especially compromised with regard to privacy. Privacy becomes one of the most consistent focuses as we follow the histories of cultural practice and ethical attentiveness from the nation's earliest days to the contemporary moment. Its consistency gives it a consequentialist value, as well as an analytical heft.

It is important to clarify the difference between the *idea* of privacy and the legal notion of a *right* to privacy. The legal right was given its most noticeable expression in an 1890 essay by Samuel Warren and Louis Brandeis in the *Harvard Law Review*.[4] Their essay, prompted by the authors' outrage over the intrusion of the press into their family lives, argued for making this kind of invasive interest a wrongful act—a tort—in the law.

The cultural context of their essay is important. This early call for a privacy tort is thoroughly engaged with matters of culture and identity— the same substance that, eighty years later, motivated the declaration of a right to privacy in constitutional law. Warren and Brandeis wrote: "Gossip is no longer the resource of the idle and of the vicious, but has become a trade, which is pursued with industry as well as effrontery. To satisfy a prurient taste the details of sexual relations are spread broadcast in the columns of the daily papers. To occupy the indolent, column upon column is filled with idle gossip, which can only be procured by intrusion upon the domestic circle."[5]

Who are those who gossip? What is the material difference in their lives, or their bodies, that makes them available for this kind of aspersion? The class presumptions of Warren and Brandeis clearly separate certain bodies from the privacies that the Boston lawyers argued as their birthright. Their rhetorical approach in making the argument was to distinguish themselves from another class of Bostonians, whose disreputable habits included their interest in the lives of the rich and famous. This issue of the invasion of class privacy was arguably the one that grated the most for the authors of "The Right to Privacy"—and that may have prompted its composition.[6]

It is important to contextualize the claim that Warren and Brandeis made, noting that the era in which they wrote was one in which women had no right of franchise and were arguably sequestered rather than sheltered within the domestic sphere, while blacks—although considered citizens by the Constitution—lived under the *Plessy v. Ferguson* doctrine of "separate but equal" that continued the segregationist policies and attitudes that had earned black bodies differential and dangerous treatment under the law for scores of years past *Plessy*.

For Warren and Brandeis, the legal idea of privacy would be most properly shaped through the law of torts—in Judge Thomas Cooley's words, "the right to be left alone."[7] From his phrasing, Warren and Brandeis argued for a right to an "inviolate personality." In order to explain the desirability of an integrated (inviolate) personhood, the authors articulated a difference between privacy and property. Property was a right that existed outside of a person—what the authors called an "incorporeal" right. Their essay suggested that privacy was an intimate aspect of identity.[8]

The legal theorist Jonathan Kahn has explained the distinction, noting that a privacy right would be "manifested in the integrity of one's individual identity or persona."[9] In fact, as Kahn reminds his readers, the first case to recognize a right to privacy, *Pavesich v. New England Life Ins. Co.* (1905), was indeed about someone's persona—the complainant sued over the right to use his image. Paolo Pavesich found his likeness published in an advertisement for the life insurance company in an Atlanta newspaper. He sued, arguing that his privacy had been compromised. The court's judgment in support of his claim structured an association between the right to liberty and the idea of a right to privacy. The court held that liberty included the right to be let alone, and that this was an entitlement to determine "one's mode of life, whether it shall be a life of publicity or of privacy." In finding for Paolo Pavesich, the Georgia Supreme Court became the first court in the nation to recognize a distinct right to privacy. The first citizen in the United States to gain this legal recognition was white and male.

There is good reason to associate the early legal frames of privacy with contemporary issues in bioethics. Kahn locates the value of privacy quite clearly in the principlist language of bioethics, when he writes of privacy "as it explicitly implicates dignity, autonomy, and the integrity of the self."[10] Engaged as well with the language of ethics is the legal scholar Anita Allen's assessment that "we promote and protect privacy to show moral respect . . . and to confer moral dignity."[11] Despite the shared residency of privacy and ethics, the idea of privacy as an ethical value is not without potential contradiction. Different values attach to privacy when the reference is to a private place, rather than to a private body or private knowledge.

If privacy means location and concealment—a private place—social history offers abundant evidence that private domestic spaces (homes) have been places where bad acts are practiced on vulnerable women. Warren and Brandeis argued specifically for the privacy of the home as a domestic space free from the intrusion of gossip or the invasions of the press. But it is specifically because of the privacy ordinarily granted to families and homes that the bad acts that happen within can be concealed from the public view. This is the argument of some feminist legal theorists, whose cautionary stance regarding privacy points to the ways that women's history indicates their specific vulnerability to domestic (home-centered) violence.[12] Although there are several considerations that fairly easily blunt the force of an argument against women's embrace of the private because of the histories of violence and hegemony, these gendered perspectives of privacy are further nuanced when race is added to the identitarian mix. Race problematizes concealment as a thoroughly pejorative space. The theorist Patricia Hill-Collins reminds her readers that black women could not even anticipate the idea of sanctuary within private family spaces. She writes that "under slavery, U.S. Black women worked without pay in the allegedly public sphere of Southern agriculture and had their family privacy routinely violated."[13] For enslaved black women, private spaces were both desired and potentially harmful. The difference of gender by itself cannot explain the cultural complexities invested in the idea of privacy.

The idea of a body's privacy includes the reasonable expectation of being free from unwanted touch and exposure. Consider the kind of wariness that parents and guardians frequently impart to youngsters about how they should consider their own bodies in terms of the touch or attention of strangers. Violations of that expectation are governed by criminal law. Underlying the ethic of this claim is the idea that a person should be able to anticipate his or her body's insular integrity. Nevertheless, despite the reasonableness of such an expectation, women's bodies have become sites for public regulations that belie those notions of integrity and insularity.

In 1890, a dispute regarding private knowledge prompted the Warren and Brandeis essay. The authors complained over the intrusive habits of the press that they wanted to render liable to tort law. In *Pavesich*, the 1905 Georgia case, the plaintiff had an expectation that his personal information (a photograph of him) should not be circulated in the public sphere without his knowledge and consent. Three years before *Pavesich*, however, New York courts overturned a similar claim made on behalf of Abigail Roberson, a minor, whose image had been used without her permission to advertise flour.[14] The language was clearly gendered in the Roberson case. In turning down her privacy claim, the court noted that the image was a flattering one, and remarked that it was reasonable to have found the company's interest in her beauty complimentary. With reference to the privacy she claimed, the court declared there was no precedent available on which to base her claim for a right to privacy. Only three years later the Georgia Supreme Court determined that it was undesirable for Paolo Pavesich to have *his* image on an advertisement. That court was able (and willing) to determine a way in which his privacy claim had standing. The matter of the desirability of the image did not reach the court's determination. Rather, the Georgia court constructed a relationship between privacy and liberty (a constitutionally enumerated right) that allowed it to rule for the plaintiff. Although other factors were probably in play, it is important to ask what difference the plaintiffs' gender might have made in the judicial review of the two cases.

In the evolution of privacy interests and rights, gender is a particularly rich area for consideration. Women are the public face of domestic violence, and women and girls are publicly seen as particularly vulnerable to sexual violence. These social indices inform contemporary public dimensions of reproductive rights issues—legal, medical, and social—and help us to understand the ways in which these private matters entered the public square accompanied by certain bodies, but not by others. U.S. history illustrates that women's fertility had an early impact on commerce and the nation's sustainability, and that other advances in our nation, especially with regard to scientific research and medical practice, tied the social judgments regarding gender to the construction of public policies. As the so-called weaker sex, women were seen as being in need of particular kinds of protections. That social perspective encouraged states to claim legislative authority in matters that involved women's bodies. Although a federal right to abortion was eventually upheld in the 1973 ruling in *Roe v. Wade*, a subsequent case, *Planned Parenthood of Southeastern Pennsylvania v. Casey*, indicated that states could assert interests that limited that right because of their protective authority over their residents. In other words, women's bodies can be associated with rights in which others might have (or claim) legal, if not ethical, interests. Is a woman's womb a private space? If so, whose?

The issues in medical ethics and law that are the focus of this chapter do not escape the gendered social histories that accompanied the evolution of privacy.[15] Consider the way in which the practices of modern gynecology depend on a U.S. medical history that included experimentation on enslaved women and girls. J. Marion Sims, a nineteenth-century physician, developed a surgical remedy for vesicovaginal fistulas[16] that depended on the availability of subjects from enslaved women. His operations were performed "openly and publicly on nude African American women, when to do so with white and middle- and upper-class women patients would have caused severe repercussions . . . Having patients who were his property or were given over completely to his authority and care gave him a carte blanche that did not apply to patients who owned their own bodies."[17]

It is clear that Sims's black patients had neither legal nor cognizable moral claims to autonomy.[18] They were enslaved, and their bodies were legally considered to be property. Warren and Brandeis's consideration of bodies as incorporeal did not apply during the days of slavery. Although there have been some modern suggestions that it would be appropriate to regard his practices as bound to the social conduct of his era, these arguments ignore the era's critiques of slavery and its vigorous abolitionist movement.[19] Sims's decision to own slaves indicates his choice between competing ethical paradigms. But it cannot be said that he was without the moral alternative that the abolitionist movement provided. The historian Marie Schwartz explains that "encounters between enslaved women and slaveholders' doctors endow the themes familiar in the historical literature on slavery . . . The importance of their wombs and breasts for the future of slavery meant that the struggle for domination centered on women's bodies. The women suffered a peculiar form of violence as slaveholders and doctors exploited female anatomy for their own purposes. Thus women experienced slavery differently from men precisely because of their childbearing experiences."[20]

Marion Sims's nineteenth-century practices mirror patterns of practice with regard to reproductive medicine in the United States, where racial disparities in notice, treatment, and outcomes persisted throughout the nineteenth and twentieth centuries and into the twenty-first.[21] Sims's conduct was an early illustration of the way in which black women's bodies acquired distinctiveness and interest—not often benign—that would follow them throughout the nation's history.

When we notice the ways in which the founding of the nation was critically attached to its interest in women's fertility and reproduction, it is difficult not to notice that this early pattern of public interest in women's reproduction eventually extended to state interests and constitutional questions. Women's individual autonomy in regard to their bodies' privacy as it specifically related to their reproductive potential has been a matter of ethical compromise shaped in part by the identity of the woman's body in question.

RACE, RIGHTS, AND REPRODUCTION

A consideration of different ethical paradigms for different bodies is the issue for some readers of the science fiction writer Octavia Butler, who disagreed with her explanation of the subject of her short story, "Bloodchild." Butler was even a bit piqued by readers who read it as a story about slavery. "It isn't," she wrote in a postscript to the story. "It's a number of other things though."[22] Its plot is fixed in an imaginary future, when humans have become the hosts that allow an alien species to reproduce. The aliens deposit their eggs for gestation inside human males or females. "Bloodchild" tells a story that leads to a human boy's decision that the alien named T'Gatoi should implant her egg in him rather than his sister. Instead of this being a story about humans enslaved to aliens, Butler declared that "Bloodchild" was her "pregnant man story."[23]

The circumstances of the humans in this short narrative—are they willing participants or drugged into acquiescence?—shape a significant part of the story line, easily explaining readers' responses to this as a story about slavery. But there is another focus in "Bloodchild," one less apparent than the tension surrounding the selection of a host for the alien's egg. The aliens control and shelter the event of birth. After they implant an egg into a human host, they attend its hatching. It is a disturbingly bloody event, in some ways not unlike a human birth. Gan, the boy who agrees to host T'Gatoi's egg, wants the privacy shield removed from these births, noting that when they go wrong, they have incredible potential to frighten humans. Gan says: "'No Terran ever sees a birth that goes right.' She looked down at me. 'It is a private thing. It has always been a private thing.' Her tone kept me from insisting—that and the knowledge that if she changed her mind, I might be the first public example. But I had planted the thought in her mind. Chances were that it would grow, and eventually she would experiment."[24]

Despite Butler's pique, it is not unreasonable to read slavery into the text of "Bloodchild." Certain events clearly evoke confinement—as when Gan's sister lies against T'Gatoi's multi-limbed body: "The whole left row of T'Gatoi's limbs closed around her, holding her loosely but securely. I had always found it comfortable to lie that way, but except for my older sister, no one else in the family liked it. They said it made them feel caged."[25] Clearly the confinement and restriction are like enslavement.

Despite these reasonable allusions, it is likely that Butler's focused interest was the generational differences between humans and the ways in which they responded to their new status in a mixed-species society that altered gender roles. In this fiction, the humans who live alongside the aliens include two generations—parents who had unsuccessfully fought the alien invasion, and their children who have grown up knowing little else but aliens and humans who live alongside each other. Butler's tentacled aliens need human children to reproduce and ensure the domination of their own species. Consider the metaphorical similarity between the aliens' interests and the interests of white doctors who attended enslaved women in the United States in order to ensure the health of their progeny, so that the vitality of the plantation system was not compromised. The history of J. Marion Sims's experimental surgeries during an era when blacks were considered less than human forms an interesting corollary to Butler's story, which blurs the lines between slavery and acquiescence and between autonomy and helplessness. How do we read the differences between the brother's and sister's decisions when we know that one or the other must host the alien egg? Is a compromised autonomy still a form of autonomy?

Even if the relationship between humans and aliens feels like capture, this narrative clearly emphasizes the younger generation's easier accommodation of alien colonization. The story explores a shift in sex roles—especially when the reader encounters the sexual intimacies between humans and aliens that are dominated by the aliens. But the unresolved issue seems to be generational. One difference between the generations, in addition to the younger generation's greater acceptance of the human role in alien reproduction, is its different understanding of what matters should be rendered public. It is not irrelevant that the implantation is described with an eroticism familiar to human sexual encounters that implicitly seems to render the scene private: "I undressed and lay down beside her . . . I felt the blind probing . . . the puncture was painless, easy. So easy going in. She undulated slowly against me . . . 'Do you care?' I asked. 'Do you care that it's me?'"[26]

After that encounter. Gan's own delicate probing of his interest in making birth a public event is the issue that remains. Does the value of privacy differ between genders and generations? Certainly the issues of privacy that have emerged with contemporary technologies trouble the traditional perspectives attached to the question.

The provocative title of Butler's story carries the full symbolic weight of the social and biological issues related to reproduction. From the intimacies it engages to matters of origin, relation, ownership, and property, a "bloodchild" underscores the complexities of reproductive biologies when the subject is a focus for science and society. The questions of justice and autonomy in this story resonate deeply with readers and probably provoke their associations of its narrative to slavery.

From a bioethical perspective, the principles of justice and autonomy are especially vital to reproductive medicine, not only because of the differential treatment that women and women of color have historically experienced and the gender- and race-based imbalances that permeate our culture, but because the history of bodies as property is closely intertwined with the principle of autonomy. These principles allow bioethics to focus on the consequential differences between women and men, the differences that emerge between women, and the policy histories within and between these differences. For each, privacy is a touchstone.

A federal, constitutional right to privacy was first articulated in *Griswold v. Connecticut*[27] and further developed in *Roe v. Wade*, the 1973 Supreme Court decision that effectively rendered decisions about maternity (within certain parameters) in the hands of women (and their physicians). The language of *Roe* and the persons it implicates merit a review of the ways in which the bioethical principles of autonomy and justice focus, in this matter, on the complex ethics of reproductive rights. According to Louis Henkin, the legal scholar Laurence Tribe considers autonomy to be deeply implicated in a "variety of rights of privacy and personhood" and believes that "the key issue in Roe is not privacy but autonomy, which Tribe defines in terms of control over one's body and reproductive destiny."[28] The intersection between privacy and autonomy that the law wants to identify might be more easily found within the ethical terrain that they share. Here, language from the Warren and Brandeis essay resonates, especially the idea of an "inviolate personality." From the perspective of bioethics, an inviolate person might be understood as one whose body is able to claim and sustain the relatedness between autonomy and privacy.

Butler's "Bloodchild," for example, is ultimately about reproduction in a landscape of humans and aliens so extraordinarily different from the norm that reproductive rights are distanced from the normatively gendered way in which we are accustomed to consider them. Does gender change these rights? Perhaps it is precisely that dramatic differentiation from the norm that allows Butler's readers to consider the ways in which privacy and autonomy are compromised, and identities rendered fluid, based on the controlling authority of the aliens. Shedding the human seems to liberate an ethical regard that is not compromised by social privilege or prejudgment. This reflection on the ethics of identity with regard to an alien body is a challenge. Another narrative, this one significantly more local and historically easier to imagine, captures within more familiar landscapes the factual social complexities that are inherent in reproduction, identity, and ethics.

WHO'S THE DADDY?

In an 1893 short story, the Southern writer Kate Chopin described a "foundling child" named Désirée, who had grown into a lovely and accomplished woman.[29] Under the tutelage of her stepmother, Madame Valmonde, Désirée achieved the goal established for socially privileged young women when she married into a venerable Louisiana plantation family. But at the story's opening, nineteenth-century readers would have noticed her anonymous origins as a foundling as a foreshadowing of the story's tragic potential. Classic symbols in the story harbinger the unhappy conclusion and support readers' suspicions. Madame Valmonde describes L'Abrie—the home that, with her marriage to Armand Aubigny, had at first welcomed Désirée—with language that emphasizes its dreariness: "The roof came down steep and black like a cow." And although the symbolic importance of the family's ancestry is folded into the description of the plantation—"big, solemn oaks grew close to it, and their thick-leaved, far-reaching branches"—the imagery that recalls the genealogical family tree also harbingers the familial tragedy that will come. Chopin writes that the plantation's arbor "shadowed it like a pall."[30]

The birth of the Aubigny first-born is narratively engaged in a way that unmistakably reminds readers of the importance of the family line and the assurance of a male heir: "Armand is the proudest father in the parish . . . chiefly because it is a boy." However, soon after Désirée's baby is born, its "color came in"[31] and indicated that the baby was a "visible admixture"[32] of white and black blood. Désirée's standing in the family, as well as her baby's, was no longer viable. "'Armand,' she called to him in a voice that must have stabbed him. 'Armand' she panted once more, clutching his arm, 'look at our child what does it mean? Tell me.' 'It means . . . that the child is not white that you are not white.' A quick conception of all that this accusation meant for her nerved her with unwonted courage to deny it. 'It is a lie; it is not true, I am white! . . . And my skin is fair,' seizing his wrist. 'Look at my hand; whiter than yours.'"[33]

Désirée's exile from the Aubigny home occurred nearly immediately after her husband affirmed her own fears with his declaration that their child "is not white": "she walked across a deserted field [and] disappeared among the reeds and willows that grew thick along the banks of the deep sluggish bayou, and she did not come back again."[34]

The fate of color and kinship seems sealed at this point in this brief story, but Chopin is not finished with her narrative. In a letter from his mother discovered after Désirée's departure (and, readers presume, her death), Armand learns that it was he, and not his wife, whose bloodline belonged "to the race that is cursed with the brand of slavery."[35] The tell-tale color that revealed the child's nonwhite lineage came from Armand's genes and was not embedded in his foundling wife's obscure origins.

The story's other twist is more subtle and comes to our attention through its publication history. When it was first published in *Vogue* in 1893, the story was titled "The Father of Désirée's Baby." But it took only a year, and the story's publication in Chopin's 1894 collection *Bayou Folk*, for the child's paternal line to disappear from the title, which became "Désirée's Baby." It is a telling absence and shift, especially when we know that the story's surprise ending will reveal narratives about race and the ethics of identity that, despite the contributory factors of a father's body and blood, are played out on women's bodies.

The "stain" of race[36] and its unavoidable attachments are a consequence of our nation's peculiar legal history. The laws of inheritance that entered state legal codes during the era of slavery, and whose social impact extended beyond that era, were written to protect white males from losing the social privilege bound to their being propertied, and their necessity was occasioned by a system of legal and social slavery that produced its own peculiar set of potential inheritors. Property laws reinforced racial hierarchies and were a direct consequence of the sexual economies of slavery. Little wonder that property and privacy would become intertwined in legal analysis, and that some scholars would find a need to distinguish them from each other.[37] But an important analysis suggests why this might not be a justifiable distinction.

The consequence of sexual expression included the evolution of controlling legal regulations that attached to the ways in which the history of differential regard of race mattered. As we see in "Désirée's Baby," even white males who were not really white earned this protection—as long as their true color was not visible. Whiteness, the property of inestimable value, forced a convoluted complex of statutory interventions.[38]

Privacy is the first apparent loss that Désirée experiences when her baby's color reveals itself. A postpartum lying-in was traditional for women of Désirée's social class. Women of another class or color would have immediately returned to their labors, a demand of the plantation economy that would contribute to the racialized assignment—and perceptions regarding the veracity—of a physiological distinction between the physical stamina of black and white women and girls. Safely cosseted within the domestic bliss of her husband's estate and waited on by silent slave women in her home, Désirée basked in the protective sanctuaries available to women of the patrician class. But in Chopin's story, once the baby's color began to reveal itself, "something in the air [was] menacing her peace." Her privacy was the first loss. Chopin writes that there were sudden "unexpected visits from far off neighbors who could hardly account for their coming. Then a strange, an awful change in her husband's manner."[39] The baby's increasingly visible race pierces the private sanctuary of their home, leaving it vulnerable to the public scrutiny of her neighbors. The story's conclusion turns on the unfairness of the discovery: it is Armand, not Désirée, who has black parentage, and therefore it was his genetic line that added the color to their child's complexion. In both literal and figurative ways, Désirée's baby is evidence of the cathexis of racialized and gendered identities, and of privacy.

One might easily limit this narrative to its early era; its social indices are certainly marked by historical distance and are certainly more legible within the lens of the past. Further, the narrative is a fiction, an imaginative construction of place, event, and character. But consider a more contemporary narrative—this one decidedly not a fiction—that illustrates the ways in which women and race have earned a particular vulnerability to public scrutiny and how "[The Father of] Désirée's Baby" was a narrative that foreshadowed our sustained investments in color as/and the body.

PUBLIC SPECTACLE AND PRIVATE KNOWLEDGE

When we consider the ideas of autonomy and justice in bioethics, legal narratives are one way to review the histories of bioethics' principles and their practices. A focus on gender narrows this terrain, and a focus on race specifies it even further. The practice of both medicine and the science that informs it has long had an association with the law that we can also draw upon in order to better understand the social circulation of ideas of privacy and the body. Legal case narratives help us to understand the social heritage of some of these claims.

In 1924, in New Rochelle, New York, Alice Jones and Leonard "Kip" Rhinelander fell in love and married. The social differences between them were stark. She was "colored" (in the language of the era), and he was white. She was from a working family, and he was from a wealthy family who were descendants of the French Huguenots. The marriage had her family's approval, but the vehement disapprobation of his. In fact, when Leonard's father learned that Alice was colored, he ordered his son to have the marriage annulled. Kip obeyed and filed a petition of annulment, based on an allegation of fraudulent contract—claiming that he did not know his wife was colored. Once the New Rochelle newspaper ran a story about their marriage with the headline "Rhinelander's Son Marries Daughter of a Colored Man,"[40] their private marriage became a public scandal.

Local and national newspapers followed the often titillating events of the trial. Alice's and Kip's love letters were read aloud, and the intimate details of their sexual activity—some of which implied intimacies that violated the sexual mores of the era—ensured that the story had a wide and interested audience. The fathers' roles in the proceedings are not insignificant, but—much like the father of Désirée's infant—the men disappear into the narrative. Kip's father controls his son's actions, even dictating the annulment process.[41] Alice's father's color is visible evidence of his daughter's lineage, even though Alice's complexion was at least light enough to sustain a court trial. She became the "body of evidence" with regard to the petition's claim of fraudulent deceit. Alice's response to the lawsuit was that she had not hidden her race from Kip.

The trial proceedings support this argument, noting that Kip had visited Alice's home, had met her father, and could not reasonably have thought otherwise of her race. The prosecution argued that her race was a private knowledge that Alice had withheld. The defense asserted that it was not only knowledge the couple shared, but that it was publicly evident in her family's visible color. The adjudication of competing claims would ordinarily involve the presentation of evidence from both sides. There would be testimony in favor of each claimant's position and legal arguments strategically devised to support the evidence. But this trial's outcome was strikingly out of the ordinary. The jury's decision inverted social expectations of race, gender, and privilege—which would have argued for Kip's success—in its holding that Alice Rhinelander had not committed fraud. Kip Rhinelander's petition for annulment was denied. An elite, white New York family lost its case to a working-class colored girl. How could such a socially incredible event occur?

The Rhinelander outcome was intimately related to how deeply, even how quixotically, significant these matters of color and discernment were to the social order. Recall that in Chopin's short story, as soon as Désirée's baby's color "came in," the fates of the mother and infant were sealed.

A visible black ancestry immediately and unalterably assigned you to the colored side of the population. As the Rhinelander case reveals, the law used that assignment to regulate society and to maintain the social orders it produced. Since rights were adjudicated in part by color, in both legal and extralegal systems, it would have been disruptive and disturbing to believe that color was not discernible and that social orders and assignments were unreliable.[42] Kip's claim could not stand. In fact, the judge gave him a medical excuse, declaring that he was "brain-tied,"[43] effectively placing him outside of the norm of the upstanding and intelligent white males who were judging his case and who could not be so easily deceived. It was "not unknown for middle class white families to explain their children's wayward behavior by accusing them, quite literally, of being insane or otherwise damaged."[44] The legal scholar Angela Onwuachi-Willig argues that the court's ruling "used basic contract and family law to reify the social construction of race" and that the case is a legal "testament . . . to societal desire by Whites for legal recognition of the idea of biological race."[45] Her point regarding the law extends as well to society and science. In that era, a reliable biology of race was one way that society stratified itself, allocated rights, and determined a person's value. The Rhinelander case is remarkable not only because of the public rehearsal of these matters, but because of the jury's decision. In other words, to support public policies, it was more important to deny Kip's annulment than to rule that Alice could have successfully concealed her color. Society's ability to distinguish between races had to be upheld. It was the appropriate public policy outcome for the era. But at what cost to privacy? Even though Alice prevailed in court, the victory was not without substantial personal consequence. Her private body was used to produce the public knowledge of her claim.

Alice never testified at her trial. She did not have to: the public spectacle of her naked body spoke for her. The primary evidence of the defense against the charge of fraud had to be that, given their intimacy, Kip could not have been ignorant of her color. His racial associations, her family, and the company they kept would support Alice's argument but would not be conclusive. To make their claim indisputable, Alice's attorneys devised what may be the most extraordinary spectacle ever entered into evidence in any courtroom in the United States. The court record details this extraordinary jurisprudential moment:

> The Court [i.e., the judge], Mr. Mills, Mr. Davis [Alice's attorney], Mr. Swinburne, the jury, the plaintiff, the defendant, her mother, Mrs. George Jones, and the stenographer left the courtroom and entered the jury room. The defendant and Mrs. Jones then withdrew to the lavatory adjoining the jury room, and, after a short time, again entered the jury room. The defendant, who was weeping, had on her underwear and a long coat. At Mr. Davis' direction she let down the coat, so that the upper portion of her body, as far down as the breast, was exposed. She then, again at Mr. Davis' direction, covered the upper part of her body and showed to the jury her bare legs, up as far as her knees. The Court, counsel, the jury and the plaintiff then re-entered the court room.[46]

Some readers may be puzzled, thinking that if it were a matter of being able to see Alice's skin color, her arms and legs would have sufficed. But there was a more intimate social expectation regarding an anticipated biology of difference at work—that her nipples and areolas would be brown rather than pink, like a white woman's—and that that revelation would win Alice's case.[47] The expectation that prompted Alice's disrobing was that private color might intimately reveal itself— even if it was not apparent in everyday public encounters. There was no need for Alice's voice here—neither her disclaimers nor her assertions. Onwuachi-Willig writes that "her body spoke for itself on the issue of race."[48] To preserve the social order that depended heavily on racial discernment in order to differentially assign rights, the jury had to rule against one of their own (the jury was all white and all male, typical of this era when women had only recently won the franchise) and return a verdict in favor of a colored girl.[49]

The attachment in this event of the social to a presumptive biology of race invigorates a particular set of beliefs about difference and identity that were apparent not only in social and community affairs, but that leaked into science and medicine as well. At the beginning of the twentieth century, the anthropologist Ernst Haeckel compared the "Negro" to "wild tribes of men" whose climbing skills were ape-like.[50] Within a decade of the Rhinelander trial, the U.S. Public Health Service would initiate its "Tuskegee Study of Untreated Syphilis in the Negro Male"— a forty-year study that would advance its scientific objectives by not treating the men who were enrolled with medication that would have ended their illness and saved their lives.[51] In 1924 Congress passed the Immigration Restrictions Act (also known as the Johnston-Reed Act), and the federal government's conditions for restricting immigration by race into the United States paralleled the rise of eugenics in U.S. policies designed to institutionalize social reforms.[52] The 1924 law barred Italians and Eastern European Jews from immigrating, labeling these populations as "dysgenic."[53] What is notable in these social and political movements is that the language attached to these social determinations is medicalized in ways that specifically evoke twinned genetic determinations about identity and value that animate legal and political processes. Diane Paul, a political scientist, writes that "to the extent that eugenic sentiment had taken hold it was used in a socio-scientific way to buttress the conventional social order and provide a scientific gloss on racial and class prejudice."[54]

Perhaps it is because of our bodies' presumptive privacy, especially in regard to sex and sexuality, that it seems appropriate that the body's exemption from public spectacle exists in relation to private (often considered home-bound) conduct. Public attention to otherwise private events, like sexual intimacy, and an ideal domestic sanctity that closet this intimacy provoke outspoken advocacy for privacy even as these kinds of intimacies seem to make the most riveting public narratives.

Especially in law and medicine, where these matters come for adjudication or diagnosis, the public narrative that attaches to private events is not without its effects on our legal systems as well as our ethical judgments. Color rendered Désirée's private life public, with the neighbors' visits in the midst of her lying-in, the gossip of slaves, and the open speculation about her body's origins and what they might mask. In legal history, the right to privacy is attached to the body's domestic conduct. In their seminal essay, Warren and Brandeis pronounce their concern that the "sacred precincts of private and domestic life" are threatened when "what is whispered in the closet shall be proclaimed from the housetops."[55]

While "Désirée's Baby" imaginatively tightens our focus on these locational concerns, the Rhinelander case makes them factually apparent. Early cases in U.S. law and medicine take up the same narrative, recognizing that women's bodies provide an especially provocative script that renders them available not only to public scrutiny, but also to private invasion. This legal and medical notice has not been accomplished without the accompanying social and historical frame of what a woman's privacy and a coordinated racial recognition might mean. Little wonder that Kate Chopin chose as her drama of race and gender in the South a narrative that would include the most titillating elements of private matters gone public—those that attach to reproduction and race.

Although *Rhinelander v. Rhinelander*'s legal argument involved a contractual issue of fraud, it had a decidedly social and familial context that turned on the presumptive biology of the body in evidence. During the trial, that context was evident in national and frenzied newspaper coverage of the story. One reason that the story had such social heft was the potential of the couple's private sexual intimacy to produce a child that would inherit the Rhinelander family's wealth. Interracial intimacy was certainly not outside of custom. But when that intimacy's consequence might attenuate white ownership of property and wealth, the law intervened. Adrienne Davis explains that "in the southern states . . . redefinitions of inheritance practices incorporated specific rules to deal with the political economy of slavery. Balancing testamentary freedom versus lineal descent of wealth and redefining chains of success were complicated by slavery's peculiar treatment of race and sexuality."[56]

The disapprobation directed toward the mixing of races focuses on adult intimacy. But it was the consequence of this mixing that merited the restricted social and legal environments of these relationships. New York State did not have statutes preventing intermarriage, but many other states had laws against both miscegenation and intermarriage. Kip Rhinelander "stood to inherit millions from his family,"[57] and—since New York had no statutory barrier—so did any children a legitimate marriage could produce. Preventing that transfer of economic property was arguably worth the public embarrassment his family might suffer in a court proceeding. The jury had to choose between sustaining the validity of social presumptions about race and difference and rendering a decision that would safeguard a particular white family's fortune. Although they chose to protect the social system and ruled for the defendant, in the process, Alice Jones Rhinelander suffered a body blow.

A CALCULUS OF RACE

Medicine's story is similarly textured with regard to gender and race. Slave women like those who are shadowy background figures in Chopin's fiction had, in fact, been subjected to the most heinous of medical experimentation. And ironically, as late as 2004, questions seem to remain among ethicists about whether or not the experiments of J. Marion Sims on anesthetized black and Irish patients were understandable given the boundaries of the times.[58]

Sims was a slave owner, and his failure to use anesthesia on the black Southern women he operated on—who were his property—and later on lower-class Irish immigrants in the North was in direct contradiction to his treatment of upper-class white women, whose constitution, he argued, was too delicate to endure surgery without the benefit of ether. The historian Martin Pernick explains that nineteenth-century surgeons commonly selected patients for anesthesia based on the belief that whites, especially white women, were more sensitive to pain than people from lower socioeconomic classes, as well as blacks and American Indians.[59] Certainly the social biases of the era made that kind of discrimination common. But consider this modern ethicist's explanation of Sims's discriminatory treatment:

> He considered his vaginal surgeries to be minor procedures and did not use anesthesia with either his African-American [sic][60] or Irish-American patients . . . However, he *found* that upper-class white women could not tolerate surgery without ether . . . Throughout his medical career Sims maintained a classbound prescription for the use of anesthesia with an unspoken premise that those women in the

wealthy tier were by far the most vulnerable to pain. To be fair, this was not untypical of practitioners in the latter 1800s.

He owned slaves in Alabama, and in fact actually purchased one or more of the slave women he experimented on . . . However he was not a virulent racist, and by all accounts treated black patients politely, if in a patriarchal fashion.[61]

What might explain this author's ethical uncertainty regarding whether Sims's conduct indicated a moral disregard for his patients? What does this modern scholar mean by asserting that Sims "found" a different level of pain tolerance in white and black patients? Legal and historic social distinctions of race, class, and gender may account for this modern explanation of Sims's experiments, but does this explanation shift our appropriate moral judgment of his conduct? Are ethical principles selectively subject to era and situation? Consider the ways in which reproduction matters in the lingering ethical questions relevant to Sims's experiments.

As noted earlier, a vesicovaginal fistula is a result of giving birth at a young age—when the mother's body is not yet mature enough to withstand the forces of labor. How did the enslaved girls that Sims operated on become pregnant? What happened to their children? Nowhere in Sims's autobiography is there a single word about what brought these enslaved girls and women to the barn on his property that he used as his operating theater. Sims's experimental population is not unlike other people from society's least privileged and protected groups—often women or blacks—who, either without giving fully informed consent or without even understanding the consequences of what experimentalists have done to them, have been subjected to unethical research practices over the years. The issue of reproduction has remained critically relevant to this research. If social or medical histories regarding poor women or women of color develop along predictable lines, should ethical judgment depend on the era in which the practices occur, or should it rely on abiding moral principles that outlast the moment?

The social judgments that underscored Sims's practices find parallels in practices with women patients in the middle of the twentieth century.

As in the Sims episode, these are also poor women of color, and the science that was being investigated would have value to reproductive medicine.

In the 1950s, a new housing development in Rio Piedras, Puerto Rico, became the site for Gregory Pincus's trial of a new birth control drug. The medical historian Laura Briggs writes that from "eugenics to population policy to sterilization . . . the sexuality and reproduction of poor women would become the battleground—symbolic and real—for the meaning of the U.S. presence in Puerto Rico."[62] Briggs summarizes the "multifaceted and rather complex story of the 'problem' of Puerto Rican reproduction in the 1920s, '30s, and '40s . . . overpopulation, eugenics, and birth control programs intervened in debates about whether the island was entitled to independence, and whether the 'race' of the island's inhabitants was 'black' or 'Spanish.'" Briggs argues that the association of the large population of poor women on the island with its "economic ills" provided the "occasion for further U.S. involvement," including the clinical trials of pharmaceuticals designed to stem population growth—what she calls foundational "postwar population control policies" that "made certain kinds of reproductive autonomy impossible for many Puerto Rican women."[63]

Convinced that large doses of progesterone would be an effective method of birth control, and unable to get a population of subjects on the U.S. mainland, Pincus and his assistants enrolled a Puerto Rican study population for trials of a new birth control drug.

Birth control would be illegal on the U.S. mainland until *Griswold v. Connecticut*, in 1965. Prior to that Supreme Court case that lifted restrictions on the exchange of information or materials regarding contraception, the Comstock Act of 1873 had made the sharing of contraceptive information illegal. This federal legislation was supported by laws in more than twenty states that banned birth control with even more restrictive language—an example of what can happen at the state level even with federal legislation as the ruling authority. As in the earliest days of the nation, the federal and state interest in the fertility of women citizens was tied to national objectives. In *New Dimensions in Women's Health*, Linda Alexander and her coauthors consider "race suicide" to be the ethic that prompted laws of the early twentieth century. Although the nation still encouraged fertility, the prescription had become more focused and particularized. The authors explain that "race suicide was an antifeminist theory developed between 1905 and 1910 in reaction to the lower birth rates and changes in family structures that were attributed to the birth control movement. President Theodore Roosevelt believed that upper-class, educated women were failing society by not having large families and that they were allowing the upper classes to be overtaken by immigrants and the poor."[64]

Linda Gordon, a historian, connects Roosevelt's support of large families to his theory that "the whole fabric of society rests upon the home." Focusing on Roosevelt's desire for people of "normal stock" to have six children and people of "better stock" to have more, Gordon explains this as a "strand of race-suicide thought—belief in large families, women's domesticity, nativism and racism . . . For Roosevelt, virile men, womanly women, and large families were necessary conditions for the world supremacy of white Americans." Roosevelt's administration politicized these beliefs, beginning with attacks on the contemporary rise in birth control rhetoric and "sound[ing] the then-fashionable eugenic rhetoric of building the 'race.'"[65]

Birth control researchers found freedom from these U.S. regulations in Puerto Rico. However, even there they cloaked their interest in contraceptives, describing their project as "family planning." Interested in the market for a viable contraceptive, the researchers continued their work even when 17 percent of the subjects in Rio Piedras complained about side effects manifesting as dizziness, nausea, and headaches. In fact, the researchers attributed the subjects' complaints to "the emotional super-activity of Puerto-Rican women"[66] and continued aggressive trials that eventually expanded to cover over four hundred Puerto Rican women. Despite one report by the researchers that "fully 65 percent of all users had complained of nausea, gastralgia, headache, dizziness, or other symptoms,"[67] the study was not moved to another location. Patient complaints did not trump the site, a "most impressive slum district . . . with scarcely room between for a squeezed pedestrian." Researchers who were eager to exploit the island's unique location and population described Puerto Rico as "crowded, impoverished and ripe for an intensive birth control program—a prototype underdeveloped country on America's own doorstep."[68] Commenting on the shift of the research from laboratory animals to human subjects, the philanthropist Katherine McCormick, writing to the birth control advocate Margaret Sanger, said that it would be necessary to find "a *cage* of ovulating females who would submit themselves to clinical experimentation."[69] Several scholars recall McCormick's comments with reference to the Rio Piedras trials.[70] Ethnicity, poverty, and gender cooperated in the development of a drug that was initially prescribed for trial participants at a dose of 300 mg a day for each dose. The researchers wanted to make certain that the drug would completely block ovulation during the period of their clinical trial. By the time the drug was marketed for public use, in 1960, perhaps with more attention to the side effects reported in the Puerto Rican trials, the Food and Drug Administration (FDA) approved its use in doses of 2.5 and 5 mg—a decrease from the clinical trials of about 98 percent. The disparity between the trial dosage and what was determined to be a safe dosage for public consumption is extraordinary. What caused the difference: medical ethics that were peculiar to gender and ethnicity, or a clinical trial in urgent pursuit of profits and, as a consequence, careless?

The early call for fertility in the United States had given way to policies that selected populations of certain women for reproductive experimentation and control, indicating the effects of political and legal views of women and minorities on public health policies. Some of the medical procedures in question were certainly elective. Nonetheless, it is important to acknowledge the fact that electing to undergo such procedures took place in the context of a public health ethic that socialized these medical matters in ways related to the social construction of race and poverty. Black and poor white women in the South did experience forced or coerced sterilization. And even after the era of Jim Crow, black women of the North and South were the focus of these state-supported medical decisions.

Women of color were vulnerable to public health decisions that involved permanent birth control—in other words, sterilization. By the time that Clarence Gamble led an "experiment in population control" from 1950 to 1958 in Trujillo Alto, Puerto Rico, "more than one-third of the women of childbearing age in Puerto Rico had been sterilized, the highest percentage in the world at the time."[71] During the 1970s on the mainland, Native American women in the West were subject to this medical procedure. Dorothy Roberts, a legal scholar, writes that "in four Indian Health Service hospitals alone, doctors performed more than 3,000 sterilizations without adequate consent between 1973 and 1976. For small Indian tribes, this policy was literally genocidal. One physician reported that '[a]ll the pureblood women of the Kaw tribe of Oklahoma have now been sterilized.'"[72]

The bioethicists Ellen Moskowitz and coauthors write:

> The United States has a sorry history of imposing permanent contraception, in the form of sterilization, on socially marginal, stigmatized, or disabled persons. From the 1920s to the 1950s, eugenic sterilizations were increasingly common, supported by the laws of most states, federal law, private eugenics groups, and some individual medical practitioners. The goal was purportedly to improve national life by preventing certain classes of people, often women who were poor and of non-European descent, from having children.[73]

The same attitudes persisted even during the years following the civil rights movement, when the sensitivity about racial disparities would seem likely to have prompted a greater focus on ethics. For instance, in 1973, Minnie and Mary Alice Relf—two sisters from Montgomery, Alabama, aged fourteen and twelve—were sterilized under the auspices of the federally funded Montgomery Community Action Agency, which offered family-planning services. Their mother had signed an X on a consent form that she thought would allow them to receive the contraceptive Depo-Provera, a drug then in clinical trials. The resulting lawsuit, *Relf v. Weinberger*, made the abuses in the system so clear that the federal government revised the regulations regarding sterilization without informed consent. It also banned the use of the procedure on the mentally incompetent and children.[74]

Nearly two decades after the Relf sisters' sterilization, a vehement national debate began, spurred by an article in the *Philadelphia Inquirer* in 1990 on the connections among population control, poverty, and long-acting contraceptives—in this case, the drug Norplant.[75] The author of the article suggested that Norplant, just approved by the FDA for public use, might be a reasonable solution to inner-city poverty, noting that "people having the most children are the ones least capable of supporting them." The furor that followed seemed to indicate that this was the first time federal officials might be connecting inner-city poverty and birth rates and creating contraceptive policies to disrupt the connection.[76]

But it was a federal agency that had led the Relf sisters to a hospital in 1973 and that indicated it had permission from their mother for the sterilization procedure, although in fact she believed that she had agreed to a long-term contraceptive. An article in *Time* regarding the sisters' sterilization sparked both outrage and approval of the procedure. *Time* reported that "shortly after the [contraceptive] drug was banned because of undesirable side effects, two nurses paid a visit to the shabby apartment where the Relfs live on $150 monthly welfare payments . . . Mrs. Minnie Lee Relf recalled that the nurses told her that her daughters—Mary Alice and Minnie—would have to go to the hospital for more shots. They said she must sign a paper, so she marked a surgical consent form with an *X*. The girls were taken to the Professional Center Hospital, kept overnight, and then sterilized the next day by tubal ligation."[77] Nonetheless, medical personnel in Alabama in 1973 came out in favor of controlling poverty and black pregnancies, just as some respondents to the *Philadelphia Inquirer*'s article would do.

There were questions about whether Mrs. Relf gave informed consent to the procedure, whether she had the legal right to consent to it, and whether the government had the right to perform the operation. The Montgomery Community Action Agency "insisted that the operation was properly explained to Mrs. Relf, but she denies this."[78] Rebecca Kluchin notes:

Perhaps the girls' sterilization constituted a genuine, albeit terrible misunderstanding between the clinic staff and the Relfs. Regardless, the neo-eugenic intent of the clinic workers' actions remains clear, as evidenced by the clinic staff's insistence that sterilization constituted an appropriate alternative to Depo-Provera for two sexually inactive preteen girls . . . Clinic records suggest that the staff did not confine this practice to the Relfs; they targeted other poor black girls whom they also predicted would bear children out of wedlock. In 1973, the Montgomery Community Action Agency sterilized eleven females. Ten of the eleven patients were black, and five, including the Relfs, were between the ages of twelve and seventeen. These records show that in the early 1970s, forced sterilization had evolved beyond the targeting of those who had born children out of wedlock; some family planning clinics had begun to sterilize "unfit" girls who, they predicted, would become unwed mothers.[79]

An ethical review might begin with an analysis of the judgments made by the staff of the Montgomery Community Action Agency, and the ethical principles they attached to their decision to sterilize twelve- and fourteen-year-old girls. Was their conduct arguably beneficent? The race of the girls and their mother seems to be a vital dimension of this story and a critical ethical dimension of similar cases, especially after the *Philadelphia Inquirer*'s article two decades past the Relfs' sterilizations.

Relf v. Weinberger noted that between 100,000 and 150,000 women had been sterilized under federal programs. Coercion was an issue— submitting to the procedure was linked to the continuation of welfare benefits. Certainly the ethical issues in this story are substantive and related to the principles of autonomy, privacy, and beneficence, as well as the gold standard of medical care: informed consent. But those issues merit an additional level of scrutiny when we review how intimately they are linked to the exposure of the women and girls' private identities. Circulation of the story in magazines like *Time* and newspapers such as the *Philadelphia Inquirer* places this intimate matter into public view. Is privacy or autonomy in this matter possible without a consideration of identity?

Norplant was approved by the FDA in the early 1990s and was marketed as an innovation in contraception. Instead of permanent birth control, or the short-acting progesterone, Norplant (and Depo-Provera) were longer-term birth control mechanisms lasting—in the case of Norplant—for up to five years. Norplant was quickly followed by the approval of Depo-Provera, a drug that had been in trials since the 1970s. Those trials were conducted on women who lived in third world countries like Nigeria, India, Costa Rica, and Kenya. In the United States, women at the Grady Medical Center in Atlanta were enrolled. Thus, black women were the predominant populations for the trials. In the United States, at Grady Medical "for eleven years, no annual reports were filed with the FDA, as required."[80] Given the large trial population and the extended length of the trials, what would have prevented an ethical review of the Grady trials?

According to Roberts, there were 4,700 black subjects in the Atlanta trials. She appropriately connects the judgments about poverty and race that link poor and black women and girls in the United States with their counterparts around the world. She notes that "the South African government under apartheid pressured Black women to use Depo-Provera by distributing free injections at factories and farms, sometimes threatening women with the loss of their jobs if they did not consent."[81] In the United States, women and girls who were welfare recipients, like the Relf sisters, were sometimes coerced into using Depo-Provera or Norplant. Each of these intrusions obviously focuses on a woman's (or girl's) reproduction, or its nullification. In these cases, the ordinary privacy expected to accompany sexual intimacy becomes a matter of government notice, regulation, and control, which are attached to particular bodies. This loss of privacy seems unique to women and specifically attached to their reproductive potential. The bioethicist George Annas notes: "The constitutional right to privacy is founded on liberty interests in intimacy and freedom of association, and notions of self-identity and self-expression. Privacy is not a technocrat's toy, and does not require the government to keep its hands off any method of procreation that inventors can devise."[82]

An important way of acknowledging the history of privacy in these practices and of considering what ethical questions are involved is to recover the associated history and public policies that might explain their vitality.[83] Fiction presumes this thick backdrop and tolerates the creative complexities that can emerge somewhat more easily there than in case studies. Fiction even makes it possible to consider why one resolution to the quiet horrors accomplished in private might lead Butler's character Gan to imagine that it would be better if alien birth were a public spectacle.

Medicine is not the only space in which rights and legal claims to privacy must be negotiated; these claims also have a fractured history of discourse among legal theorists.[84] Despite the differing analyses and conclusions, privacy seems nonetheless the tie that binds the legal to the medical, and both of them to the social. When Davis traces the "Private Law of Race and Sex" in the antebellum era, she notes that the obligatory relationships that private law governed also determined "which relationships will give rise to enforceable (or permissible) obligations, and which ones will not." She recalls an important category of distinction that judges of this era brought to questions of inheritance: "the sexual relationships . . . formed under slavery ought to yield succession rights to estates." These were claims of "inheritable blood."[85]

This is the subtext of Chopin's postbellum story. Her readers would have included whites who had good reason to be concerned about their own inheritance and difficult-to-trace family lines. When "the Father of . . ." falls away from the title, the bodies left for public scrutiny are the woman's and the child's, suggesting that as long as normative privileges of heterosexuality and whiteness are not interrupted (and the story's outcome assures us that they will not be), men's secrets will retain their presumptive privacy. In "Désirée's Baby," the surprise discovery at the story's end does not change Armand's material condition. He is still alive, wealthy, and publicly white[86] because he has exercised the authoritative control over his circumstances that comes from his social and racial standing.

VISIBLE ERROR AND HERITABLE BLOOD

In May 1998, one couple's effort to have a baby with in vitro fertilization (IVF) technology was unsuccessful. The eggs that Deborah Perry-Rogers received during the procedure did not attach themselves to her uterus. But on the same day, and at the same clinic, another couple's effort was doubly successful. Twin sons were eventually born to Donna Fasano. Deborah Perry-Rogers sued for custody of one of them.

In-vitro fertilization—in which the egg and sperm are fertilized outside of a woman's body—is a modern process that has antecedents in history. Artificial insemination proceeded the era of IVF. The first recorded artificial insemination in the United States was described in a 1909 article in *Medical World* by a physician named Addison Davis Hard. The article reports an event in 1884, when William Pancoast, a Philadelphia doctor, procured a semen sample from the "best-looking" of the class of medical students who were observing his examination of an anesthetized patient. Using a syringe, he inserted the semen into the woman's uterus. A pregnancy later resulted for this patient, who had come to Pancoast for treatment of infertility. She did not know what had happened to her during anesthesia—in fact, it was a secret that was not revealed until twenty-five years later, upon the publication of the *Medical World* article. Scholars have speculated that Hard was the sperm donor as well as one of the student observers of Pancoast's unethical procedure. Elaine May, who retells this story, notes it as the first recorded artificial insemination from donor sperm, but "not necessarily the first that occurred."[87]

In April 1998, Donna Fasano was celebrating the success of her IVF procedure. The fertilized eggs that had been implanted had both attached themselves to her womb. But the pregnancy that resulted would soon become a legal, if not an ethical, quandary. Deborah Perry-Rogers was also a patient of the clinic, and her ultimately unsuccessful procedure happened on the same date. The next month, the embryologist responsible for the egg transfer admitted to the clinic physicians that he had used a catheter for embryo transfer that contained the fertilized eggs of the Rogerses while implanting the Fasano eggs. The clinic notified both women of the procedural error. By that time Donna Fasano was carrying twins. However, only one of the eggs successfully implanted in her womb was hers. The other was the fertilized egg of Deborah Perry-Rogers. The clinic urged the Fasanos to undergo DNA tests as well as amniocentesis. But Donna Fasano agreed only to a DNA test four months after her twins were born. In December, she gave birth to two boys of visibly different races.

It was not the first time such an error had occurred in an IVF procedure—but it was an unusual occasion because the error would be visible. So what ethical or legal difference does race make?

In 1993 in Holland, Tuen and Koen were twin sons born to Wilma Stuart, a white woman who lived in Utrecht. Stuart had been a patient at a fertility clinic in that city, and her white husband, Willem, had donated sperm for her procedure on the same day that a black West Indian man had donated sperm. When Stuart's twins were born, one was visibly white, the other black. Stuart's response to the error reveals a good deal about society and race. "When I learned the truth I felt as if I had been raped," she said. The social reading of this error continues in a newspaper article: "By the time the twins were two years old the difference was startling . . . When they took the boys to a zoo Willem says they received more attention than the animals." The article notes that "at least twice before, parents have been the all-too-apparent victims of heartrending IVF mix-ups."[88] It is of course absolutely reasonable to suspect that there have been scores of other errors like this. But notice the way in which race seems to change the language and the kind of attention this particular error receives. The social attention to racially visible IVF error occasions not only heightened medical and legal scrutiny, but public notice of the error.

Court documents reveal that the Fasanos did not act on their knowledge of the medical error until Deborah Perry-Rogers, who had learned of it, located the Fasanos and filed a suit to determine the genetic background of the brown-skinned Fasano twin. DNA testing confirmed that Joseph Fasano (named Akeil by the Rogerses) was the genetic child of Deborah and Robert Rogers.[89]

This dispute has become widely discussed in legal and medical literature in a way similar to the focus of "Désirée's Baby"—as a maternal crisis. How do the stories that engage the conflict become narratives about maternity? Whose autonomy is at issue, and whom does justice view as the ethical subject? The public presentation of the case reveals the way in which the mothers become the focus and the fathers drop out of the calculus, much as Armand is removed from Chopin's story, and race becomes the inescapable background. After the New York State

Supreme Court rule that declared the custody of Akeil Rogers should be remanded to his biological parents, the majority of states (with the exception of California) have traditionally considered the birth mother, or gestational mother, rather than the genetic mother, to be the legal mother. When courts cannot rule based on the best interest of the child, they are left to make a decision on the basis of a maternity that has already exceeded the traditional boundaries. In the dispute between the biological and gestational mothers, the New York State Supreme Court ruled for the genetic mother despite the history of case law that would have focused on intent and the gestational mother. The legal theorist Leslie Bender bases her analysis of the decision on the essentialism assigned to geneticism as opposed to nurtured relationships:

> The tendency of courts [is] to default to a genetic essentialism . . . when trying to unravel the complicated messes of maternity created by mistakes in ARTs [assisted reproductive technologies] . . . Genetic essentialism asserts that our genes and our DNA are the essence, the core, the most important constituent part of who we are as human beings; therefore genetics should overpower any other factor when defining biological parenthood. Genetic essentialism reduces human beings to the contents of our cells. It ignores the ways our cells and environments interrelate, the ways our physiological system functions as a whole organism, and the ways our minds and hearts affect our being. Additionally, genetic essentialism renders all our ways of nurturing and being nurtured by one another for naught.[90]

What were the contours of this case that caused this shift from precedent? The following case offers one explanation.

Stephanie Harnicher gave birth to triplets, and in the course of treating one of them for an illness, blood tests revealed that the child was not biologically related to George Harnicher or to the sperm donor chosen by the Harnichers.[91] The Harnichers' physician had chosen to use micromanipulation of Stephanie Harnicher's ova with the objective of increasing the potential for fertilization. Donor sperm was included with George Harnicher's sperm to increase that potential as well. The Harnichers had selected a donor whose physical characteristics were similar to George's.

The Harnichers brought suit for medical malpractice after discovering that two of their triplets were not related to George or to the selected donor. The legal claim was based on emotional injury, arguing that the "disappointment in the results of the donor mix-up has resulted in mental illness accompanied by physical symptoms."[92] The Utah State Supreme Court denied their claim, holding that there was no triable issue of fact regarding bodily harm. The error is similar to the one in *Perry-Rogers v. Fasano*: the University of Utah was found to have used sperm that did not come from the donor who had been selected. But what ethical questions emerge with the consequences of this error? Here is no contest over parenthood—no other family claiming a child as their own, which was what happened in *Perry-Rogers v. Fasano*. The issues in the Harnicher case do, however, raise important questions regarding who is the appropriate subject of our ethical focus. The mother? The father? The triplets? The medical clinic? Since the legal claim was brought against the university that owned the clinic, does the question of justice embrace bioethics' principle of autonomy—or is this an opportunity to review the distinction between the court's public system and the body's private law?

Certainly the extraordinarily intimate matters of sexual relationships, sexual dysfunction, and personal health become topics for adjudication in disputes such as this. Is it because reproduction is seen as a women's issue that the court record reflects a greater emphasis on Stephanie Harnicher's claim than on her husband's? In its decision, the court writes: "The Harnichers do not allege that the triplets are unhealthy, deformed, or deficient in any way. Nor do they claim any racial or ethnic mismatch between the triplets and their parents."[93] Notice the court's rhetorically parallel association of deficiency with racial and ethnic mismatch. It seems that a visible error with regard to race or ethnicity shifts the calculus of harm.

Racial visibility can actually move ethical and legal judgments away from precedent and establish a new set of practices particular to identity. In these cases, contradictory judgments are evident when race matters. Legal analysis has only recently instituted a doctrinal basis for cases of reproductive dispute, based on the doctrine *mater est quam gestatio demonstrate* (the mother is demonstrated by gestation). Despite the Latin name, the doctrine is nearly as recent as the disputes that have emerged around new reproductive technologies.[94] It does, nevertheless, indicate the way in which doctrine emerges from social issues that have deeply complex, even contradictory, histories.

There would seem to be little need to establish a legal claim regarding maternity were it not for the reproductive technologies and surrogacy that complicate the ways in which motherhood might be achieved. The errors and missteps that might accompany these practices are legend — but many of them are also invisible, until and unless genetic analysis steps into the picture. The kind of analysis that the Fasanos eventually used to determine the genetic background of their twins emerged only because of the public visibility of the clinic's error.

In July 2002, an article reported that a "white IVF couple have black twins." In that case, "the white mother wants to keep the babies, according to the UK's *Sun* newspaper, but a black couple is also believed to be involved."[95] Evidently unproblematic pregnancies and births that result from technology such as this have no need for genetic analysis. Case law reveals its contradictions here and makes it clear that the decisions of who should be awarded custody of a disputed child ultimately have social origins. Even in bioethics, the principles of justice seem conflicted when race matters. In both of these disciplines, a woman's privacy is an encumbrance, if it is not simply ignored.

The relationship between individuals is a matter for what is called private law — generally expressed as torts and contracts. The legal scholar Adrienne Davis is correct to point us toward private law as the legal site where these claims begin to inhabit bodies that are recognizable to the rest of us. So when the legal scholar and theorist Dorothy Roberts argues that a "relationship between the practice of medicine and social order"[96] begins with a consideration of women of color, she actually is considering a legal relationship that is understood under the doctrines of private law. Private law and concerns about privacy and identity meet in ways that engage our social histories of race and gender. In Chopin's tale, color — even the presumption of color other than whiteness — dramatically changes the landscape. Women quite literally bear the evidence that will determine their social status. Their vulnerability seems to begin with their reproductive potential and to conclude with the state's interest in the outcome of that process.

Roberts argues that the interrogation of women's bodies starts with women of color, noting that "poor women of color have never enjoyed a private protective relationship with their doctors."[97] Although the domestic sphere is the first place in which private, sexual conduct occurs, the relationship of women to their physicians, and to the medical profession in general, is a second, significant site where privacy matters for women, especially—given this nation's history—for women of color. Roberts's claim can reasonably be extended to an argument that women cannot enjoy a private or protective relationship with their own bodies because of the way in which they are inevitably and consistently subjected to legal and medical scrutiny. Reproductive potential stands in opposition to privacy in both of these forums. Consider the breach of privacy that lies in a conduct too many of us too easily engage in: reaching out to touch a woman's pregnant body, and noticing or commenting on her pregnancy, even if she is a stranger. What social determinations make a woman's visibly pregnant body publicly available to a stranger's touch? We might consider here the differences in treatment between Sims's white and black women patients who were experiencing complications of childbirth or medical issues attached to their pregnancies, and the spectacle of his operations:

> When Sims undertook his fistula experiments . . . "women's doctors" averted their eyes in a chivalrous fashion as they knelt to tend to the modestly clothed ladies of their class . . . However, Sims, working with enslaved blacks, was constrained by no such delicacy. He made the women undress completely, then kneel on hands and knees while he and several physicians took turns inserting a special speculum he had devised to open the women's vaginas fully to view. "I saw everything as no man had seen before," marveled Sims. Montgomery physicians flocked to Sims's shack to see what no man had seen before. So did prominent citizens and local apprentices.[98]

Bioethics' interest in reproduction arguably begins with legal cases that asserted a woman's right of choice. The rights associated with the

Roe decision, whether deployed as an issue of choice or as one of privacy, foreground a particular kind of claim as well as the criticism that *Roe* should not have located the right to privacy in the liberty clause of the Fourteenth Amendment. The history of court decisions that involved women and reproduction and that intersected with a privacy right began in 1965 when, in *Griswold v. Connecticut,* the Supreme Court declared unconstitutional laws that prohibited the use and distribution of contraceptives. This decision gave women unfettered access to contraceptives, regardless of their marital status. In the case, Estelle Griswold, a physician, ran the Planned Parenthood League of Connecticut and provided contraceptives to married women. In an opinion by Justice William O. Douglas, the court declared a fundamental right to privacy, protected under the liberty of the due process clause. The domestic scenery in the narrative of his decision is important. Douglas wrote: "Would we allow the police to search the sacred precincts of the marital bedrooms for telltale signs of the use of contraceptives? The very idea is repulsive to the notions of privacy surrounding the marriage relationship."[99]

The language in *Griswold* recalls the language of Warren and Brandeis, who had also written about the sacred precincts of the home: "The common law has always recognized a man's house as his castle, impregnable, often, even to its own officers engaged in the execution of its command. Shall the courts thus close the front entrance to constituted authority, and open wide the back door to idle or prurient curiosity?"[100] Today the gendered bias in this language is blatantly evident—a bias reasonably underscored in some liberal feminist arguments against a privacy right—and makes clear the ways in which a right to privacy traditionally and historically has allowed men to commit bad acts against the women in their homes. One might add to this mix the privacy that protected hate groups—such as the Ku Klux Klan—in their commission of violence against minorities. Hidden behind white sheets, or beneath tented masks in more contemporary versions, privacy can easily become a dangerous space if we consider it as a shield that protects those who engage in heinous acts. Are these histories appropriately addressed with a declaration that privacy is against the interests of women and minority groups, and therefore should not be available? The legal scholar Anita

Allen responds to arguments regarding privacy and gender that would give safety priority over privacy: "Male hegemony is not a reason to reject the idea of privacy and the private sphere. Absent radical social reorganization, to reject the private sphere is virtually to reject the notion of reliable opportunities for seclusion, anonymity and solitude."[101] The ethical principle of autonomy that arguably contains much of the apparatus of privacy seems differentially valued when identity is matched with autonomy.

In *Eisenstadt v. Baird*, a decision subsequent to *Griswold*, the Supreme Court declared unconstitutional a Massachusetts law that prohibited unmarried people from receiving contraceptives. Following a lecture on birth control at Boston University, William Baird had given Emco contraceptive foam to a woman. The Court's decision was based on the law's disparate impact—the fact that married persons could receive contraceptives, but unmarried persons could not. Justice William J. Brennan Jr.'s language is telling in terms of the Court's focus: "If the right of privacy means anything, it is the right of the individual, married or single, to be free from unwarranted governmental intrusion into matters so fundamentally affecting a person as the decision whether to bear or beget a child."[102] Note that the series of decisions concerning reproductive rights for women were all domestically situated, within the marital space, the home space, or our intimate imaginaries around sexual acts. The government paradoxically identifies these matters as private at the same time that it determines it has a legitimate interest in their adjudication.

The legal argument that the gestational mother is also the legal mother (*mater est quam gestatio demonstrat*) appeared first in U.S. law in 1983 and is related to the "longstanding *pater est* presumption"—that the father is demonstrated by marriage.[103] For the last several decades, jurisprudence seems to have followed a guideline that is tied to an arguably ethical principle of autonomy—that the birth mother is also the legal mother. Mason and McCall Smith underscore the importance of this principle, arguing that "no genetic niceties should obscure the fact that [gestation and birth] are the essential features of motherhood."[104] The "birth rule"—*mater est quam gestatio demonstrat*—has operated as a determination of maternity. Courts that have used the guideline of *gestatio* have also connected their decisions to the more legally robust contractual position of intent—that is, a determination of what was the intentional outcome of the technology, or surrogacy, used by the parties in dispute.

But what happens when there is a mistake? Error in these events is not generally evident. Only with DNA testing can the biological relations become certain. However, the visible difference of a black child born to white parents, or the reverse, makes the error immediately evident. Intent is an efficient solution, and the legal precedent of gestatio seems a stable basis for a claim. But both fail when private errors enter the public domain.

Although these cases seem to create usable legal precedents, the ethical principles of justice, autonomy, and non-maleficence are still in use, absent an apparent standard that governs legal questions or ethical determinations. Stable doctrines or principles are difficult to establish when identity disrupts the narratives. One benefit of technology may be that it can reveal the complex personhood that lies within these contemporary cases. What establishes the ethical standing of the sperm donor? The fertilized egg? The unborn child? Does the standing depend on a noticeable or an inherited social identity? Do legal and ethical considerations of justice differ? In the cases of error, there is no intent to be considered in reaching a decision, as error is unintentional. The appropriate legal framework to apply when intent is displaced by identity is unclear.

In bioethics, privacy operates most vigorously within the principles of autonomy and justice. Although legal privacy has a specialized interpretation in the discipline of law, ethics and privacy are inclusive of the legal and reach beyond the law. If, for example, a court determines that a narrow question is at issue—such as the question of bodily harm in the form of mental illness experienced by George and Stephanie Harnicher as a result of the clinic's error—its ruling will not address the ethical questions of justice that might emerge from the case. What is the ethical status of a sperm donor? Donors frequently disappear from these narratives, as the legal and ethical questions focus on women's bodies. Recall how the father of Désirée's baby disappears from the narrative, and Désirée is left to experience the consequences of racism. But sometimes donors add another body into the mix. The experience of a surrogate makes ethical judgments regarding autonomy and justice even more of an ethical conundrum.

PRIVATE BODIES

Because *private* can mean hidden as well as intimate, privacy is an idea that simultaneously has complex, even contradictory, uses. A private space might be one protected from view because of a benign—that is, a harmless—intimacy, expressed as a neutral social value. The harm of privacy, perhaps best articulated in this ethical context as the maleficent desires of a privacy that would conceal bad acts and that would interfere with another person's selfhood, does not seem to diminish the social regard and value attached to the idea of an inviolable or private personhood. That autonomous self is engaged and practiced in the privacies of knowledge, body, and space. But because privacy is also represented in legal and social histories as a normative value and is very much implicated in the matters we value and attach to ourselves, it is a desired ethical status that is expressly evident in our value of autonomy. What happens when our own bodies' desires can only be fulfilled with another body? A final narrative, this story earlier than those already shared, might illustrate this ethical quandary.

Recall that in the Rhinelander case, the conflict between Alice and Kip was represented as a contractual dispute—specifically, the complaining party, Kip, alleged that Alice had entered into a knowingly fraudulent agreement with him. With regard to the IVF clinic errors, the legal system looked for a solution in contract law's determination of intent in order to reach a just resolution of a conflict. Even if the social histories of the parties do not bear this out, contract law presumes an equitable arrangement between parties, and the possibility of a meeting of the minds, a legal perspective that at least implies a parallelism between the parties. Bioethics' interest in the subjects' standing might find a useful precedent in an Old Testament story.

Hagar bore a child for her owners, Abraham and Sarah (a practice that was not unique to this biblical couple). Hagar's status (her standing in the matter) betrays her vulnerability and indicates that there could not have been equitable contract between her and Abraham—in fact, neither of the women stood as social equals to Abraham. But Hagar was the least of these, instructed—and given no choice, it seems—to go to Abraham, get pregnant, and then give her child to her owner and his wife. Surrogacy illustrates the ethical questions that emerge when reproduction is a right that becomes negotiable.

A *Newsweek* story called surrogacy "an act of love, but also a financial transaction, that brings people together like this."[105] "Love" is a thick description to bring to an understanding of surrogacy—and its emotive use makes a clinical narrative about surrogacy nearly impossible. Surrogacy is, as the magazine story indicates, a financial transaction as well as a legal one. The latter sphere offers quite specific ways to address disputed outcomes and participants who might change their minds. But legal review presumes equity between the contracting parties. How does bioethics consider equity? The principle of justice seems most relevant to the determination. But how does a gestational body equitably negotiate between autonomous agents who all have moral status, but who might also display competing claims and desires?

Is each party comparatively autonomous, or does a surrogacy contract render one's autonomy inequitable? Does gestational surrogacy—where the genetics is controlled by the intended parents, who contribute the egg or sperm—differ from traditional surrogacy, where the surrogate's egg and the male's sperm are combined? Does commercial surrogacy, which is banned in some U.S. states but allowed in India (for example), differ from altruistic surrogacy, where there are no payments except to cover the medical fees? Is altruism a deceptive category in bioethics? What was Hagar's obligation with her gift—the altruistic donation of her child? Hagar's identity—she was an Egyptian slave, a colored woman— was not insignificant to her status and power in the biblical story.

In some ways, Hagar's position was not much different from those of the brother and sister who could carry the alien egg in Butler's "Bloodchild." They could no more control their own reproductive potentials in the confines of the ruling aliens than could Hagar in the confines of slavery. Considering Sarah's status in that Old Testament story might help us to understand how readers receive "Bloodchild" as a story about slavery instead of one about a pregnant man.

Kate Chopin's "Désirée's Baby" could be interpreted as a narrative about the ethical dilemma of agency (autonomy) and privacy. Chopin's story was set in the plantation era—a time and locale where slavery formed the critical narrative background to the politics of color and family that brought Désirée to her tragic end. In each of these fictions, as well as in the historical moment when Alice Rhinelander found her body on public display, the ethic of autonomy and its embrace of privacy and the body's politics are deeply entwined. Is it the potential of women to bear children that renders their bodies immediately and irretrievably public and available? What makes black bodies circulate differently in these narratives? The histories of and in our bodies are, in fact, its stories and ours—and also society's mirror of its habits and traditions. Michel de Certeau has written that our society "is defined by stories . . . by citations of stories, and by the interminable recitation of stories."[106] His consideration of narrative helps us to understand the ways in which narratives and stories excavate bioethics' complex environment. Just as legal history must eventually separate persons from the idea and claims of property, literary fictions reveal their embeddedness in our cultural and aesthetic traditions. Critical histories in words, practice, and law accompany the nation's ethics of persons—its *bio*ethics.

TWO

Cartographies of Desire

In mapping the human genome, scientists performed a function that is both extraordinarily modern and as old as human history: tracing our human blueprint.
The destinations of our curiosity, the reach of our explorations, and the landscapes we encounter depend on the narrative that frames our journeys. The idea
of a map is a consistent and reliable vehicle for us to use in communicating the
discovery of this new terrain. This chapter begins with a consideration of map
making, and how that industry—whether we trace and map our families or our
genomes—is called upon to give a familiar contour to new frontiers of science.
Maps connect very different kinds of landscapes, and this chapter's interest in genomics, cloning, disease patterns, ancestry, and indigenous rights engages these
varied terrains. Our interest in privacy and identity will forge pathways through
these "cartographies of desire."

• • •

Cartography is an art that demands as much creativity, vision, and imagination (with the full emphasis on that word's genesis from "image") as it
does scientific rigor and analytical capacity. The cartographer's product
commands a particularly focused consideration from its readers. Writers
of both fiction and nonfiction have employed the allure and the attentiveness required by a map as a way of getting a high level of attention
from their readers.

Desire is an emotion that expresses the want of something or somebody. In both the industry of mapping and the texture of desire lies an

expression of longing. And in both a cartographer's effort to specify a place and a person's deep desire for some external thing or body, the need for the other is implicit, either as a knowledgeable spectator or as the wanted object.

Cartography structures (or regulates) ways of seeing and understanding. So when genomics used the idea of a map as the visual explanation for the accomplishment of sequencing the human genome, it was a regulation of our understanding of the project. In the 1990s, the Human Genome Project's (HGP) objective was to discover a single reference human genomic sequence. Although 99.9 percent[1] of the genetic data of all human beings is the same—identical genes in identical chromosomal orders—the 0.1 percent difference fuels an industry of investigations and desire. The differences appear as alleles (coding sequences within our genes) that can matter in terms of individual variations—including morphological difference, or phenotype; differences between populations; and genetic variations that produce certain diseases and illnesses. This chapter will consider issues in genomics that emerge when privacy and ethics are considered in the context of those three areas: categories of identity, population and geography, and medicine.

In March 2000, Dr. Francis Collins, director of the National Human Genome Research Institute, and Dr. J. Craig Venter, president and chief scientific officer of Celera Genomics Corporation, announced that they had completed "an initial" sequencing of the human genome. Using language that clearly suggested the cartographic shape of the project, President Bill Clinton called it "the genetic blueprint for human beings."[2] President Clinton's announcement was deeply invested in the symbolic idea of cartography. He began his remarks with a comparison of the project's achievement to a map that Thomas Jefferson received from Meriwether Lewis's expedition "across the American frontier."[3] In his comparison, this genetic map became the newest frontier and therefore, according to Prime Minister Tony Blair, available as "common property." Collins used descriptive language appropriate to his corporate interests, noting that the genome was "our shared inheritance."[4]

The White House press release celebrated the occasion as a "starting point for a new era of genetic medicine" and ensured that the public-policy frame of this research would protect corporate desires, indicating that genetic discoveries would have the oversight of patent law, a "policy of intellectual property protection [that] will promote rapid conversion of basic knowledge into useful applications . . . allowing a maximum free flow of basic scientific information."[5] The White House also acknowledged the privacy implications of the project, noting that "today's announcement builds on the Clinton-Gore administration's strong commitment to protecting *private* genetic information" (emphasis added).[6] The text reveals the irony of the political grandstanding as it underscores the potential conflict between the public and private spheres. In proclaiming that the genetic information from the project would be assured the "maximum free flow" within intellectual property considerations, a private person's ownership of his or her own genetic data is effectively dismissed.[7] Although the private sector's interest is protected in this policy statement, the interest of private persons—who will actually provide the substantive matter of the research—is not granted the same level of protection.[8] Underscoring the regulatory structure of this new era, the HGP's website includes links to the various "maps" of the human genome's sequence data.[9]

Patterns of human genetic variation can be traced through single nucleotide polymorphisms (SNPs, pronounced "snips"), deviations in genetic sequences that are not random and that occur as combinations (blocks) of alleles that are transmitted together from parent to child. The International Haplotype Mapping Project (HapMap), formed after the HGP sequenced the human genome, has adopted the metaphorical power of the idea of cartography in naming its research paradigm. Scientists involved in HapMap chart human genetic similarities and differences from participating donors from four continents. After getting DNA samples from these donors, the scientists work to identify and map chromosomal regions where genetic variations are shared. The project's goal is to discover correspondences between a map of these variants and patterns of disease, suggesting pharmaceutical and environmental factors in disease treatment and development. HapMap scientists have agreed that their information will be released into the public domain, noting that individuals cannot be identified from their DNA after the initial evaluation of their samples. The HGP paid attention to the ethical, legal, and social implications (ELSI) of the data, devoting 10 percent of its funding to address matters in science, medicine, and society associated with the mapping that might have ethical implications. The scientists were correct to anticipate that the publication of information that revealed the cellular bases of human difference would be read into existing social narratives—specifically those that animated perspectives and understandings of gender and race, as well as those that assigned to our bodies a set of differential values depending on a body's political presence and social privilege.

It might seem that we risk reducing these projects' extraordinary scientific accomplishments by comparing them to fiction. But in its frequent use of a visual map to introduce a story—whether a genealogy of characters or an illustration of routes traveled in the story—fiction reveals how a map brings a particular perspective into visual relief. This is especially true when a book of fiction has a page of maps that precedes any of the text. Readers are alerted that the narrative that follows is in part a travelogue. This prefatory visual indicator will help readers follow the story's progress.[10] And readers will be in a position to follow a particular journey with the map's fanciful[11] representation of an imagined topography. However creative these introductory illustrations[12] might be—in their markings of terrains, pathways, and populations—they are are inevitably and immediately recognizable as a map.

Consider another locative guide that exists in fiction as well as in fact. In fiction we use a genealogical diagram, or family tree, to discover the relationship of one character to another; these are famously necessary in many Russian novels, and helpful in the work of William Faulkner as well. In this book, we are similarly looking to fix the location of some character within the network of an often dense story. This kind of map— a genealogy—seems a particularly useful device to illustrate the ways in which private bodies and public texts produce a relationship between cartography, desire, and the body. Cartography structures, orders, and regulates something that is otherwise unwieldy or unknown. Desire, as our longing and our want, is itself metaphysically unwieldy, existing in relationship to its object as well as substantively being the object. Like a genealogy, a cartography of desire is regulatory—its locative effort places things or people into relationships with others.

Consequently, our reference to the discovery of the sequence of DNA as a map of the human genome not only constructs a locative project, but also produces a particularly selective representation of the illustration's relational data. This map gives the most intimate detail possible about the most minute matter of our bodies—the constitution and sequence of our DNA—specifically the 0.1 percent where distinctions between individuals lie. Genomic differences can occur within the DNA sequence or in its structure as rearrangements, insertions, or deletions.[13] When we assign significance—social, scientific, medical, or a combination of these—to the differences, they gain informational value. When genetic differences between persons and groups are interpreted within social or scientific frames, it means that our judgments about place and identity contribute to the way in which we receive and interpret information that the genomic sequences have made available. The public text that emerges from these maps regulates the ways in which we value, understand, and interact with knowledge regarding the body's most interior, most private matter. Our private bodies' implicit public vulnerability explains in part why scientists from the National Institutes of Health (NIH) who oversaw the human genomics project, as well as the author of the White House press release were careful to include (respectively) notes on ethics and privacy in their announcements of this new genomic era.[14]

Reviewing the history of our nation's laws makes it strikingly apparent that the only bodies that have not consistently experienced the stigma of identity in this country—that have not been subjected as a group to invidious discrimination, rendered a suspect class, excluded from a jury, or denied access to the ballot box—are those of heterosexual white males. Other bodies—whether they belong to women or to men who are indigenous Americans, Americans of Asian ancestry, or America's black and brown citizens—have all been specifically targeted during some period in U.S. history for discriminatory social and legal treatment. It is no surprise, then, that when a body is determined to have value, and when our desires circulate around the identities we have attached to certain bodies, the social history of identity is wedded to its calculus. Although a fiction might incorporate as its text the fact that the value of a body (or its parts) is a human condition, the historical patterns in a body's commodification are illustrated in the facts of U.S. sociocultural and legal experience.

LOCATION AND LINEAGE

In Kazuo Ishiguro's *Never Let Me Go*, Kathy H., the protagonist, is an adult when she begins to search for the site of her childhood education, the elite boarding school called Hailsham.[15] Despite meandering drives through the valleys of the English countryside, she fails to find it. The narrative indicates its elusiveness: "I might pass the corner of a misty field, or see part of a large house in the distance as I come down the side of a valley, even a particular arrangement of poplar trees up on a hillside, and I'll think: 'Maybe that's it! I've found it! This actually is Hailsham.' Then I see it's impossible and I go on driving, my thoughts drifting on."[16]

While still at the school, Kathy's friend Ruth engages in a parallel search. Ruth's was not a quest for a place, but rather for somebody. She was among the most intent of Hailsham's students in the search for their genetic origins, the humans who created them as clones. Of all the children at Hailsham, especially those who wonder about their "possible"—as the mystery human body that was responsible for their existence comes to be known—Ruth is the one who comes nearest to the discovery. It happens on a side street in the village of Norfolk. The students who had undertaken this journey of self-discovery stop with Ruth after a report that her possible had been sighted working in an office. The students gather into a tight cluster on the street corner across from the office building where they believe the possible may be at work. Ishiguro is careful to map the layout for the reader, whose gaze is as transfixed as the Hailsham students'. They stand looking into a building with an expansive front of windows, through which they see "a large open-plan room with maybe a dozen desks arranged in irregular L-patterns. There were the potted palms . . . shiny machines and swooping desk lamps. 'So which one's the possible?' 'There. Over in that corner. In the blue outfit' . . . [I]t wasn't obvious, but the longer we kept looking the more it seemed he had something . . . especially when she was finishing her laugh with a shake of her head, [it] had more than a hint of Ruth about it."[17]

Never Let Me Go is a story that intertwines the desire for place and person. There is a mystery attached to Hailsham. Readers are initially seduced into joining Kathy's effort to locate her childhood school. But the story's buried tease is that the mystery does not lie in where the elite boarding school might be, and that discovering its location will not explain the troubling undertone of the story. Instead, readers eventually learn that it is what Hailsham's students are that is the substance of trouble in this haunting novel. They, and others who are boarded in schools that lack Hailsham's cachet but fulfill the same purpose, grow up to be "carers" or "donors"—and the reader is left to slowly unravel the horror attached to these adulthood occupations. There are no private spaces of retreat or sanctuary. In fact, Ishiguro makes an issue of the loss of the private. Kathy recalls, "When I found myself alone, I'd stop and look for a view—out of a window, say, or through a doorway into a room—any view so long as there were no people in it. I did this so that I could, for a few seconds at least, create the illusion the place wasn't crawling with students, but that instead Hailsham was this quiet, tranquil house where I lived."[18] *Never Let Me Go* does not go into details about how the Hailsham children were created. But the silent question of the children's origin is a subtle subtext of the story. Some readers, in an effort to fill in the silences evident in this gap, might recall the sterile laboratory of Aldous Huxley's *Brave New World*:

> "I shall begin at the beginning," . . . the more zealous students recorded his intention . . . "These," he waved his hand, "are the incubators." And opening an insulated door he showed them racks upon racks of numbered test-tubes. "The week's supply of ova." . . . [A]nd here he . . . spoke first, of course, of its surgical introduction—the operation undergone voluntarily for the good of Society . . .
>
> "After which they are sent down to the Embryo Store." . . .
>
> And opening a door Mr. Foster led the way down a staircase into the basement . . .

"Embryos are like photograph film," said Mr. Foster waggishly . . . "They can only stand red light."

And in effect the sultry darkness into which the students now followed him was visible and crimson, like the darkness of closed eyes on a summer's afternoon. The bulging flanks of row on receding row and tier above tier of bottles glinted with innumerable rubies, and among the rubies moved the dim red spectres of men and women . . . The hum and rattle of machinery faintly stirred the air.[19]

Although Huxley's is a narrative that lays out a very specific kind of terrain, Ishiguro offers no explanatory origin story, no Huxley-like visitation of the spectral scene of "the beginning." Instead, his narrative begins years past its characters' origin, opening when they are school-aged and taught by guardian-teachers who gently ease the students into their unavoidable destinies. The story focuses on their potential: cloned children grow mature enough to be available to provide body parts for wealthy humans (the students' possibles) who purchased them anticipating the day they would need a reliable, and exactly matched, organ donor to extend their own lives. These were people privileged enough to be able to afford this extension of their own lives, even if it was to be accomplished at the cost of "completing"[20] a clone's body. In other words, the socially privileged matter of their desire had been literally inscribed onto the students—clones who remained available and even willing to donate tissue or organs until they "completed" their own bodies' potential.

This textured and troubling tale depends on the exquisitely spare narration that Ishiguro deploys to reveal its terror. What lies within the novel's mystery is so disturbing that the story, nearly as bucolic in locale as it is serene in its telling, seems the only possible device that will not interrupt the reader's growing horror. As Kathy H. and her friends focus on recalling their school days, their adult occupations seem nearly ordinary, even when they come to a realization of how they were "told and not told"[21] of their destiny. This navigation between sense and silence installs a melancholy undercurrent of sorrow and trepidation into Ishiguro's novel. A terrible destiny is inevitable for the Hailsham clones, and despite the reader's possible desire, they don't protest their potential.

The complex story is finally and simply just told. Ishiguro's fiction of the rituals, routines, and desires of their school days seems nearly ordinary; nevertheless, it is also a "version of Britain that might have existed by the late 20th century if just one or two things had gone differently on the scientific front."[22]

Although a map might be designed to lead us to a particular location, that place, like Hailsham, can be elusive. A map simply lays out the terrain in which we might find our place. *Never Let Me Go* explores a world with purposeful, corporately[23] inclined, and ethically bereft genomic intervention. Technology has been deployed to sustain human life. In this fiction, the genomic enterprise that makes human clones possible is the unspoken scientific linchpin of a public policy that the socially privileged have shaped to satisfy their desire for longevity. The novel creates a world where information is controlled by privilege as much as it is by science. In this fiction, the idea of property—as it has in the earlier history of the English-speaking world—once again extends to the body. The public's desire for the other means a body's literal consumption. The surreal aspect of this story is that its modern-day version of cannibalism is accomplished in a setting so pristine and normal that it nearly obscures the ethical abyss. The current disputes and disposition of genomic science suggest that this is only barely a fiction—only a breath away from "just one or two things . . . gone differently" in genomic science and policy. The relationship between genomics and identity—especially the genomic science that is transferred to the practice of medicine—makes the fiction of *Never Let Me Go* disturbingly credible. This is no tale of an unimaginable future. Perhaps this is why the first page of Ishiguro's 2005 narrative contains just three words: "England, late 1990s." The opening, spare and austere in appearance, is anything but that in consequence. Instead of the dramatically imagined futures that Orwell's *1984* or Huxley's *Brave New World* produced, Ishiguro dates his story in a near past—refusing to allow its displacement into an unknown era. Readers cannot look away from the story's ultimate horror, in the glimpse it offers of a dim but disturbingly discernible era. In fact, evidence indicates that we have already entered its borderlands in our own treacherous terrain of the trade in human organs. Instead of vulnerable, empathetic clones that look exactly like their human possibles, the nonfictional narratives of organ matching lead to vulnerable humans whose bodies are, in fact, merchandise. Ishiguro's fictional representation is one example of the trade in human organs that maps out across the world and that is attached to a private person's social value. But another example is the way in which the idea of kinship has been altered by genomic science—producing both enterprise and occupation in a new corporate version of human relatedness.

BLOOD BROTHERS

Although we might reasonably anticipate that in the twenty-first century, race and ethnicity will come to matter less than they have in centuries past, in fact the terrain has changed its shape, but not its subject. This is a publicly acclaimed era of privacy-ensured DNA ancestral searches, and corporately funded Genographic Projects. DNA advances in biomedical science are designed to make individualized medicine eventually available to every citizen. This goal seems to place an inherent value on the bioethics principles of autonomy—foregrounding both patient and an idea of privacy that is intimately attached to the individual's body. But if we reach the objective of individualized medicine through a narrative replete with socially determined racialisms, can the process interfere with its goal?

In an acknowledgment of the ways in which the histories of race entered the genome project's efforts, the sociologist Jenny Reardon described the competing histories within the Human Genome Diversity Project. In summarizing the shift from an engagement with race to a "genetic study of human populations," Reardon explains that population geneticists

> did critique some concepts of race [but] they also argued for the importance of others . . . A "concept of race" proved vital to the biologist's effort to create "an understanding of how our species has evolved." [I]nstead of replacing race . . . many geneticists and anthropologists interested in the genetic study of human evolution merely

believed that race needed to be reformed and refined in the wake of abuses by eugenicists, white supremacists, and Nazis . . . [L]eading evolutionary biologists . . . believed that only by demonstrating the relevance of population analysis to an understanding of the formation of races would population genetics gain acceptance within evolutionary biology.[24]

As Reardon illustrated in her narrative regarding the process of the scientists' debates regarding the vocabularies and concepts of race and populations, our historical narratives about race and our ways of seeing the world accompany us into the constitution and deployment of these new technologies.

The National Geographic Society's Genographic Project is designed to attract the public's altruism and to anticipate our desire to join the esteemed organization's corporate project to fill in the blanks on a map that will trace the earliest migrations of the human family. It is a cartographic mission. The society's website promises that participants will "gain insight into their deep ancestral migratory route, discovering who they are and how *we are all related*" (emphasis added).[25] If this seems an alluring prospect, it has, with this one appeal, met a critical objective: the Genographic Project is designed to convey a sense of urgency. Appealing to the human instinct to survive, the website intrinsically encourages a concern that without our participation in the project, the evidence of human origins will go missing: the genetic samples "from the world's remaining indigenous peoples . . . are quickly vanishing into a 21st century global melting pot."[26] The website essentially creates an opposition between its public narrative of "the" human family, and the way in which this story might be retrieved (before it is too late): through our private contributions of DNA. Participants are promised that they will be informed of their unique identities. And they are left as well with the confidence that their altruistic contribution of DNA might contribute to the rescue of our tenuous location in the grand narrative of the human family's journey.

The Genographic Project promises that participants will experience this discovery in as private a way as possible. The website's "note on privacy" assures a "confidential participant ID number" for each respondent.[27] Its promise that participants will discover their relatedness to each other stands in opposition to its procedural claim of privacy. Researchers claim the value of genomics and the mapping of DNA and locations of genetic markers lie in their intimate application; they will ultimately contribute to medicine's goal of individualized therapies—those that best match a patient's unique genetic profile. The public's contribution to the discovery of the human family's origin has a particular and very private destination. But the ethical questions arise with the disposition of the information retrieved from public volunteers.

It is critical to understand that just because a new scientific age has dawned, with the promise of keeping privacy intact and with the motivating romance of the "human family" narrative that DNA might recover, the boundaries of consensual public information and what we have understood to be private have not been resolved. Instead, those boundaries might have acquired another layer of complication in terms of what is accessible under particular scenarios. In most cases, as with the Genographic Project, it is true that companies that volunteer to locate your lineage increase the size of their own databases, and consequently the value of these databases, with each sample they receive. The cheek swab that each private person contributes is destroyed. Once the information is extracted and analyzed, the sample is rendered moot.

But how confidential is the rest of the process? Is it absolutely and unalterably separable from an autonomous private identity? A promise by a private party to keep something confidential doesn't operate as a restraint on any governmental entity held to have a legitimate interest in the information. And it also seems to be true that the promise of confidentiality has little effect on private parties who seek the information through a legal process.

One analogy that comes to mind is the case of reporters who promise their sources that their identity will be kept confidential. Reporters have professional rules of ethics that mandate this confidentiality and a constitutional protection (freedom of the press) that would seem to ensure it. But neither these professional rules nor the First Amendment have final sway when a court decides the information does not violate constitutional protection and is necessary to the legal process.[28] How many cheek swabs would these ancestry investigators actually receive if it were clear to prospective contributors that their privacy extends only as far as the government's interest, or lack thereof?

This question is of particular interest to people of color because the reinscription of racial categories that have such a fractured history in the United States has become both a product and a process of the genomic sciences. Despite the National Geographic Society's claim that we are all one human family, the privacy promises of ancestral searches, and disclaimers that race or ethnicity is not discoverable or even significant to genomic science, modern sciences are read into old scripts that are extraordinarily difficult to displace. In fact, the narrative of race actually informs some contemporary genomic science. Racialized data quickly enter the public realm and, despite the protests of some, are of interest to others. Perhaps not surprisingly, countervailing information about race and its utility is readily available, even among the specialists in genomic science. Noting that in the United States, public health's categorizations of population health risks by race and ethnicity have produced a "surveillance practice . . . that is virtually unique in the world," Richard Cooper and his colleagues argue: "Genes are regularly proposed as the cause [of a disease] when no genetic data have been obtained, and the social and biologic factors remain hopelessly confounded . . . The correlation between the use of unsupported genetic inferences and the social standing of a group is glaring evidence of bias and demonstrates how race is used both to categorize and to rank order subpopulations. Not only are the relevant genetic data absent, but the distribution of polygenic phenotypes does not suggest race is a useful category."[29]

To explain the potential effects of a single variable, Cooper and his colleagues use height as a distinction that might appear within a distribution of heritable traits, and describes what happens when variables are identified within heritable traits: "if that [height] complexity is multiplied by thousands of traits, which are randomly distributed among groups within continents, one gets an idea of the limitations of race as a classification scheme. It is nearly impossible to separate our private interest in ancestry from a public science that makes race, ancestry, and genetic information correspond and that feeds this correspondence into historical narratives that differentially attach social values based on features of identity."[30]

The contradiction between these scientists' perspectives on the significance of racial markers is not rooted in the superiority of one methodology or theory over another, but rather in the social text that generates, structures, and then fuels the interest in connecting race and ethnicity to particular genomic markers. Searching for distinctions that matter is evidence of prior judgment that distinctive information has explanatory power or value that will contribute to our knowledge.

Whether the subject is disease patterns in medicine, DNA forensic technologies, pharmacology, or recreational information about ancestry, the DNA gathering that begins the process has its source in a single human being. Even the first mapping of human DNA had its source in a single volunteer's molecular matter. Craig Venter, then president of Celera (the company that partnered with the NIH to map the human genome), used his own DNA to accomplish the historic decoding. He later published his gene map, an act that at least symbolically rendered DNA a subject for the public realm. So whether the information that is retrieved and processed as Huxley's Mr. Foster imagined, for "the good of Society" or, as Ishiguro imagined, for the benefit of the socially privileged, in fiction and in fact, the source is a private person's body.

What ethical questions emerge when we rename "race" as "ancestry" in these DNA genealogical searches, or as "populations" or "geography" in genomic investigations? One way of evaluating the ethical landscape is to consider the consequences of representing science as objective, even though it has a substantial base of social determinations. The representation of scientific objectivity essentially removes things that are labeled as "science" from certain kinds of inquiry. If particular sets of questions are suppressed because of the way in which we have categorized a field as objective, when it is, in fact, subjectively organized, the data that emerge from that field are related to its conceptual frames. This is the way in which "scientific" theories of race emerged in the nineteenth century that associated everything from skin color to the shape of one's forehead to social hierarchies of civilization that valued European descent. Consider the ways in which geography is a contemporary frame of an ancient configuration.[31]

Specialists have made arbitrary and political choices (like deciding where Asia begins and Europe ends) when identifying continental masses in one way rather than another. What happens to our explanations of migratory patterns of "groups" when the earth beneath them was differently configured than it is today? How do our desired outcomes (e.g., "we are all related") shape the input of data? When tracing and determining human migratory routes, computational specialists make certain judgments about waterways, agricultural sites, and epidemics in the analysis and input of data into systems that determine global migratory patterns. These judgments are arbitrary and are not free from social determinations. The sociologist Troy Duster writes:

> Researchers must make many untested assumptions in using these contemporary groups to stand in for populations from centuries ago representing a continent or an ethnic or tribal group. To construct tractable mathematical models and computer programs, researchers make many assumptions about ancient migrations, reproductive practices and the demographic effects of historical events such as plagues and famines. Furthermore, in many cases, genetic variants cannot distinguish among tribes or national groups because the groups are too similar, so geneticists are on thin ice telling people that they do or don't have ancestors from a particular people.[32]

When investigations begin with language that is racialized or that specifically ties into ethnicity or population, as does the language of geographically assigned DNA databases that focus on European or African ancestry, it is difficult to erase and sometimes difficult to identify the social assumptions that are carried from these texts to the data. Nevertheless, social presumptions that are present at the project's origin are indeed tied to the result.

In the Ishiguro novel, one of the reasons that the clones of Hailsham display little resistance to their destiny is that predetermination has great social strength. At Hailsham, the language of destiny was so carefully controlled that a private desire for anything different was publicly constrained. One of the guardian-teachers, in a moment of literalism that the students did not often hear, told them this directly: "You've got to know and know properly. None of you will go to America. None of you will be film stars. And none of you will be working in supermarkets . . . Your lives are set out for you. You'll become adults, then before you're old, before you're even middle-aged, you'll start to donate your vital organs. That's what each of you was created to do."[33]

The response of her students to her "outburst" was: "Well so what? We already knew all that."[34]

Science and medicine have historic intersections with social and racial presumptions. Producing new knowledge is inevitably linked to old paradigms. Does a new science discard the paradigms and start anew? Is this even possible, when the history in our words is linguistically inescapable? Reardon perceptively engages this point, drawing an important reference to Foucault's concept of biopower and noting that our "modern age witnessed the entanglement of rules that govern what can count as knowledge with rules that determine which human lives can be lived."[35] The consequences of biopower are represented in the extreme in the eugenics movement, in the presumptions and practices that motivated clinical research on Jewish children and adults in concentration camps during the Second World War, and in the pathologization and sterilization of poor and minority women in the United States. The problems with these extremes are easily noticed; more difficult to see are those cases that fall short of the extreme and that may even seem at first glance to be beneficent. Within race-based medical presumptions are those relating particular diseases to certain ethnic populations—cystic fibrosis to whites, a genetic breast cancer mutation (in BRCA1 and BRCA2)[36] and propensity for ovarian cancer to Ashkenazi Jewish women, and sickle cell anemia to black populations. Once those associations are made, research within those population groups follow in spite of the examples of nonwhites getting cystic fibrosis, non-Jews and men with those particular genetic mutations that lead to breast cancer, and sickle cell anemia in people who are not members of "black" populations but who do reside in malarial zones. Each of the social histories that have attached to these identities compromises autonomous choice. The identity receives the attention that the individual loses in the competing social narratives.

Racial identity is a positive variable in disease treatment and research. Investigations of new drugs, for example, have been attached to groups that have more social and political power.[37] One descriptor for sickle cell disease (black race) selected over another (malarial zone residence) might establish one research paradigm and undercut another. Issues of sex and gender also emerge. The association of BRCA1 and BRCA2 mutations to prostate cancer stands in contrast to the absence of public attention about genetic testing in men. This is especially apparent when compared to the public attention dedicated to genetic testing in women and girls for these mutations. In fact, BRCA mutations are publicly understood as relevant to women, despite the significance this genetic mutation might have for men. A new era of genomic knowledge and a recreational thread for DNA research does not erase the histories of disease associations that connect social identity and biology. In fact, histories of medical and social practices that have constructed certain populations as aggregate remain coherent in much of this research.

The ways in which racial and ethnic terminologies are linked to genetic predispositions illustrate another consequence of the language we choose to represent the science. Consider the shared vocabulary of urgency in the Genographic Project in particular, and in genetic medicine in general. Keith Wailoo and Stephen Pemberton perceptively note that vocabulary in the latter, pointing out that "the hype surrounding innovations like gene therapy is fueled by a powerful notion that has defined American medicine for much of the past century: the notion that we are always on the verge of a major breakthrough in the treatment of deadly disease."[38] The promise of genomic information that our human legacy will survive necessarily creates for itself a present in which that future might have potential. We become wedded to the requisites of contemporary financing and corporate investment in genomic technologies—even those that are recreational—so that our present might allow the promise of genomics to emerge.

The ideas of urgency, eminent breakthrough, the danger of lost opportunity, and the pity of a vanished ancestry gone astray because of our unwillingness to act quickly and generously are constitutive of this effort, and each shares the characteristic of pushing past a particular response in the absence of a careful, considered, public review. Privacy is persistently disappeared within the urgency of national medical narratives, especially those regarding bioterrorism and its threats. The consequence of losing particular dimensions of privacy without public notice and review because the matter is too pressing to stop to do this kind of analysis, because the information is too important, or because it has been volunteered is not inconsequential. The process is also procedurally irregular in its avoidance of the kind of detailed principled consideration that should be applied to each innovation.

On the one hand, the rarified nature of modern science removes it from lay review. Science has traditionally claimed to be too esoteric for public consumption. On the other hand, there is a vigorous narrative regarding the importance of public access to the modern science in DNA ancestry tests. Companies like the Personal Genome Project promise to publish the complete genomes and medical records of several volunteers, in order to promote research into personalized medicine.[39] Scientists who advocate public genomics argue that their clients want to "participate in a personal revolution and to make investments" in their future.[40] Genomic science's attachment to racial categories that have significant social formations is a critical indicator of a vigorous social complication in scientific advances regarding the public utilities of DNA.[41]

This is not only a particularly privileged kind of private consumption, but it also contributes to criticism that privacy concerns are standing in the way of scientific innovation. A new vocabulary peppers meetings of genealogical societies—"mitochondrial DNA" or "Y-chromosome analyses"—making it appear as if there is some expertise that attaches to the users of these terms in ways that transfer the specialist privileges associated with science to the speakers. Traditional hierarchies that place scientific knowledge above other forms of knowledge make science even more alluring. When the public interrogation and determination of medical policies (like quarantine) are subverted because the issue is deemed to be urgent, or when scientific knowledge displaces social knowledge, bioethicists—who have particular interests in the distribution of justice and in the nonmaleficence of public policies—have a considerable stake in the public representation and uses of this science.

In the current proliferation and public appeal of DNA searches—whether as a means of discovering ancestral lineages or for public policing—categories of human beings, either as populations or as ethnicities, are reified in the process. Despite the significance we attach to discovering our personal location on a branch of the human family tree, families map complex routes to the present that social policies and practices of an era deeply affect.[42] The variables in these migrations are not rendered moot, even by as unifying an enterprise as the Genographic Project. Although the kinds of analyses that reify biologies of difference might produce a romantic human family narrative, the technology transfers that inevitably come with scientific innovation produce utilities that are not quite so benign and that quickly separate privacy from a social good. In fact, the ways in which some companies are urging publication of these data sets the stage for a legal argument of common and ordinary use.

FUNCTION CREEP

One day in 2004, Steven Turner, then a doctoral candidate at the University of Virginia, was bicycling across the historic campus that Thomas Jefferson designed. Turner had no idea that he was riding straight into a controversy that would not only link him in an odd way to the university's founder, but that would also propel him into a controversy over the legacy of the slave history that Jefferson and Monticello represented.

Turner was stopped by Charlottesville police officers who were undertaking a DNA sweep, (also called a "blooding") and was asked to volunteer a cheek swab. He had been profiled—targeted because someone thought he looked like a composite drawing of an African American man suspected of sexual assault. Charlottesville police asked 197 black men to "voluntarily" submit a sample of their DNA, and 187 consented. Turner, who adamantly refused the "request," described the conditions of what would have been his voluntary consent. Turner recalled that "they kept asking, they kept asking. They said since you will not provide a sample we are going to come to your classes, sit in on them, make sure you really are a student here. I think they're harassing people, they're intimidating people. I think they're obtaining DNA under duress."[43]

In the last years of the twentieth century, DNA tests were used to link the descendants of Sally Hemings, a slave on Jefferson's Monticello plantation, to the University of Virginia's founder.[44] The outcry from Jefferson's other descendants—who protested, parsed, and otherwise challenged the test results—indicated how fragile the ideas of black and white relationships still were. When Steven Turner found himself a victim of a DNA sweep—a forensic use of the same technology that had established the undesirable kinship between "white" and "black" Jefferson descendants—he experienced racial profiling at the hands of modern science. Black citizens of Charlottesville were outraged by this police sweep for suspects. Neither the white descendants of Jefferson who protested the genetic kinship of Hemings's descendants, nor the black citizens of Charlottesville who were corralled into a sweep because of the presumption that somewhere within them would be a genetic match, felt a romantic desire for kinship.

It is important to note that although DNA ancestry searches promise to dispose of the samples, for the purposes of criminology, the actual samples are vitally significant to meet chain of custody standards for evidence in criminal trials. Police dragnets were not unique to Charlottesville. They have been used in cities across the United States as well as in England (where they originated) and Canada.[45] There is a federal dimension to DNA forensics in the United States as well. In 2005 the Bush administration proposed adding juvenile offenders and adults who had been arrested but not convicted to the Federal Bureau of Investigation's national DNA database, CODIS (which stands for Combined DNA Index System).[46] The federal database would not include the actual samples, but states would be responsible for keeping the actual samples of blood or saliva—or whatever body material had been obtained. The samples can be searched and indexed for genetic markers that could indicate phenotype, hair color, and other visible features. And they could include genetic material that was not purposefully given—either volunteered or compelled.

That kind of material is known in criminology as "abandoned DNA"—

samples that are casually and unintentionally separated from the donor. Abandoned DNA poses a particularly interesting legal matter because what we might otherwise presume—that our daily biological debris is covered under our right to privacy—does not extend to genetic data that is unintentionally discarded. We have no autonomy over this discarded material, and if we use history as a guide, the material's potential significance to our receiving a just outcome from a process—perhaps legal, perhaps related to medical insurance—is affected by the bodies in question.

Our everyday living leaves a trail of genetic evidence, cells that are shed as a part of our bodies' normal cycles. These can be found on utensils we use to eat and glasses and cups we drink from, in our hairbrushes and combs, on tissues and water bottles. The legal scholar Elizabeth Joh suggests that the collection and forensic use of this material be considered under the rubric of "covert involuntary DNA sampling,"[47] and she underscores the critical vulnerability of involuntary sampling, quoting Judge Alex Kozinski's dissent in the *United States v. Kincade*, a Ninth Circuit case about whether a parolee can be forced to provide a DNA sample for CODIS: "We can't go anywhere without leaving a bread-crumb trail of identifying DNA matter. If we have no legitimate expectation of privacy in such bodily material, what possible impediment can there be to having the government collect what we leave behind, extract its DNA signature and enhance CODIS to include everyone?"[48]

Given the pattern of the courts' deference to law enforcement, or findings that support these investigative methods, as well as the existence of CODIS—which could be expanded—what are the consequences to privacy of allowing those methods to go unregulated, and who are most vulnerable to privacy's attenuation? How does justice escape the body?

The historic links between race and crime in the United States fuel much of the anxiety attached to DNA sweeps for criminal investigation. The anxiety is not unwarranted. DNA sequence data can have multiple meanings as well as applications. Industry has aggressively marketed tests designed to ferret out the information that clients are most interested in discovering. DNA Witness uses markers that reveal physical characteristics. DNA Print Genomics uses a similar set of markers. It has clients in law enforcement as well as in ancestral searches, and its technologies were used to generate the narrative "discoveries" in the first episodes of the 2007 PBS series *African American Lives,* which revealed DNA-ancestry test results of a prestigious group of African Americans. It is not insignificant that the technologies in police profiling are nearly identical to those used to in ancestry searches. Although the argument that police investigators collect "junk DNA" that is useless for procedures more complex than the morphological markers some investigations use to narrow their search to suspects of a certain race or ethnicity, the rapid advance of this science and the samples' increasing utilities suggest this is not the case. "Some markers now thought to be meaningless may be (and have been) found to contain predictive medical information as the science progresses,"[49] and collected samples may serve a criminal sweep as easily as they might serve an ancestry search or give medical information. Watch carefully as police procedure moves to collecting DNA samples on felony arrests and not just felony convictions. The lack of public scrutiny of this shift of privacy procedures, especially as it affects certain populations of persons more aggressively than others, is notable.

The ways in which associations of race and criminality already lead to a persistent social stereotype can invigorate race-based DNA sweeps and lead to predicting criminality. Scientists already use race as a variable in tissue repositories, and there is certainly an audience for such a potential use. For all of its exaggerated drama and visual effects, the 2002 film *Minority Report* had a hint of authenticity. It is set in our legislative and juridical heartland—Washington, D.C.—in the year 2054, where a special police "pre-crime" department apprehends criminals before they have committed the crime that a group of psychics have seen committed in the future.[50] In *Minority Report,* the "pre-crime" unit captures this science's potential and offers a disturbing context for imagining the fully developed utility of what seems today just the early era of DNA technologies.

The troubling histories of categories that designate race, nations, populations, and ethnicities and of the public's use of these categories do not disappear or render themselves benign because we are just searching for our ancestors. The databases and maps are enriched with each cheek swab, and they earn their keep through their multiple and potential public and private uses. Their viability lies in extracting as much information from them as possible, not in whether or not the contractual promise to keep your ancestry a secret only you know is in fact kept.

When Ishiguro's Hailsham students are "told and not told" what will happen to them as adults, it means that they have some awareness of and complicity in their futures; they have participated at least to the degree that they have failed to rebel. Hailsham, however, is a fiction. But our own donation of DNA for one purpose invigorates the idea of the viability of DNA analyses within a complex terrain of potential uses. In fact, it invigorates that potential by enriching the database even as privacy is eroded in the process.

ONE DROP

Rick Kittles, a genetic scientist who provided expertise for the first episodes of *African American Lives*, was also a project coordinator for the African American Hereditary Prostate Cancer Study in 2000. The diverse network of specialists who worked on this study—including statistical geneticists, urologists, nurses, and oncologists—are a "model for genetics research on the African American community."[51] Ethicists are not included in the list of those who lent their expertise to the project, but Kittles's self-described "excitement at finding a family who fit the stringent criteria for study participation"[52] indicates why they might have been helpful to the effort.

"Trying to convince" a seventy-eight-year-old man who was dying of prostate cancer to enroll in the project, made Kittles, whose grandfather had recently died of the disease, recall his own loss. It would be difficult not to be empathetic at this moment, as the face-to-face professional encounter between the scientist and the patient reached intimately into the scientist's family memory. However, the bond he was there to establish was not to his own experience, but to the patient's family, in which four other men had been diagnosed with the disease. Perhaps it was this mix of the personal with the professional that led to the odd description of the meeting. Kittles was dismayed when the man "abruptly" asked: "What will this project do for me?"[53]

The moment does indeed require a pause. Although Kittles answers by reminding "him about his family" and emphasizes that "finding predisposing genes for prostate cancer might lead to the development of better drugs and treatment and genetic screening tests,"[54] a reader might wonder why the man's inquiry would have been perceived as abrupt. It seems reasonable that Kittles might have anticipated such a question. Most patients would want to understand, and many would want to hope that enrolling in a study for a disease that was slowly killing them might have some benefit for them.

This brief narrative regarding Kittles's encounter with a potential participant in a disease-based study describes a potential ethical conflict between the project's interest in an expanded database of patients, and an elderly man's privacy during the last days of his life. The vocabulary that Kittles uses to relate the encounter is important and telling. Noting that he "was preparing to *deal with* questions from [the man's] family about the study" (emphasis added) and describing the man's question as abrupt suggests a somewhat adversarial posture—pitting a scientist from a younger generation, whose professional accomplishments will ideally serve a larger public, against an elderly patient and his family, who are interested in this one private man's diminishing days of life.

This patient's usefulness for the study occurred because of a relationship between racial identity and disease. We do not know whether it was a researcher's notice of the patient, the patient's self-identification, or a physician's judgment that placed him into that racial group, but it is apparent that he was an appropriate candidate for enrollment because he was ill with prostate cancer, and because he was black.

In the United States, racial identity has a history that is bonded with blood. One drop of black blood—one ancestor in a person's lineage who was black—was often the legal standard for determining who was eligible for the rights and privileges reserved to whites, and unavailable to people of color.[55] It would not be unreasonable to anticipate that the twenty-first century has done away with this legal notice of blood identity. However, a series of twenty-first century legal decisions indicate an odd perseverance of blood-based determinations that effectively (if unintentionally) sustain science's and medicine's notice of racial categories.

In 2005, the Ninth Circuit upheld a Hawaiian school district's admissions preference for "Native" Hawaiians. Those citizens who can attest that they have at least one ancestor (born before 1959) who is a blood relative of the indigenous Polynesians who settled the islands have preferential admission to the prestigious Kamehameha schools. Legal "strict-scrutiny" was applied by the court in its holding that the schools' selective admissions policy had a legitimate remedial objective because of the systematic "exclusion and marginalization of Native Hawaiians."[56] Although the language of the decision does not indicate how Native Hawaiian ancestry might be determined, the preferential policy that the courts have declared legitimate is certainly a blood test—a court-approved remedy for past discrimination.[57]

The *Kamehameha* ruling is, in fact, a twenty-first century version of a one-drop designation, one that takes into consideration a percentage of Polynesian ancestry. In this case, the courts have underwritten the legality of a genetic claim and ensured that this particular way of tracking identity would be viable for many years to come. One could certainly argue that this is an ethical use of a genetics-based claim in its beneficent recognition of these particular citizens and the acknowledgment of their ties to a precolonial history. But consider as well bioethics' principled investment in the idea of justice. How important is the fact that blood-based legal decisions are inconsistent and subject to different public-policy goals and outcomes? Is legal notice and determination different from a medical researcher's notice? In another case that involved native rights, a group of indigenous American tribes did *not* want DNA analysis to proceed.

Kimberly Tallbear's recitation of the dispute regarding Kennewick Man illustrates the central claims.[58] In 1996 two boys discovered skeletal remains on the banks of the Columbia River in Washington State, and an initial examination of the remains determined that they could be nearly 9,000 years old. The scientists who led the investigation wanted to classify "the Ancient One"[59] as other than Native American in order to allow their research to continue, rather than have to return the skeleton to an indigenous tribe for reburial as directed by a 1990 federal law, the Native American Graves Protection and Repatriation Act (NAGPRA).

The U.S. Army Corps of Engineers, which controlled the land around the Columbia River where the skeleton was found, had jurisdiction and planned to follow the dictates of NAGPRA. But before this could be done, eight anthropologists sued the corps for ownership of the skeleton. They thought its value to science—the remains were believed to be the oldest ever found in the Americas—was especially significant. Their lawsuit requested permission to date the skeleton by radiocarbon dating and to subject its organic material to DNA analysis in order to determine its genetic identity. The federal court that finally ruled on the dispute determined the remains were properly governed under earlier legislation (the 1979 Archaeological Resources Protection Act), which would correspond with the scientific community's claims. Further, the court indicated that the remains were not culturally identifiable—so indigenous American tribes' claims that the skeletal remains were their "Ancient One" were not upheld. The court allowed DNA analyses to proceed against the wishes of the other litigants. The critical policy matter that emerges from this dispute is that those analyses could eventually verify theories that connect genetic identity to geographic origin and then to property (land) claims (specifically, the Bering Strait theory).[60]

When a body becomes a specimen, whatever its age, it loses the presumptive privacy and regard ordinarily due to a deceased human.[61] Rituals of conduct—including burial rituals and ethical standards for the treatment of the dead—are fairly rigid regarding the deference due to the dead, and desecration of a body is a criminal act in most jurisdictions. So at what point does regard for a human's bodily privacy shift to a concern for the public knowledge available from that body—or its DNA? Does death change the boundaries of a body's privacy? The Genographic Project's seemingly benign, and narratively compelling, goal of discovering how "we are all related" is accomplished by reducing contemporary claims for individual privacy in favor of a corporate contribution to the project's knowledge base, and the project's consequences are decidedly less romantic than the discovery of human kinship might imply. Citing the Indigenous Peoples Council on Biocolonialism, Tallbear observes that the Kennewick Man controversy is a good example of "how human genetic diversity research may be used to authoritatively contradict indigenous claims to identity and rights over human remains."[62] Tallbear quotes Debra Harry and Frank Dukepoo's explanation that "scientists expect to reconstruct the history of the world's populations by studying genetic variation to determine patterns of human migration. In North America, this research will likely result in the validation of the Bering Strait theory. It's possible that these new 'scientific findings'. . . can be used to challenge aboriginal rights to territory, resources and self-determination . . . [T]he United States has long recognized archetypal matching as legitimate techniques for establishing individual identity."[63] The Kennewick saga and the Kamehameha schools' selection of its students illustrate that the assignment of legal identity and the legal constitution of a DNA-based claim are not without legal, social, and political consequences. The genetic goal of establishing a relationship is not simply a story of kinfolk—it is deeply penetrated by ethical judgments. In her critique of the Genographic Project, Tallbear leaves her readers with a provocative conclusion regarding a narrative's destination, as well as its location:

> By getting caught up in scientific debates about the truthfulness of molecular origin stories, we cede the intellectual and moral authority to scientists. We enter their territory and give them the opportunity to render our world views as untruths, to demean our power . . . [W]e should be working . . . to make sure that . . . our stories are heard as clearly as those of anthropologists and geneticists when the state acts to influence our lives . . . Or rather, that our stories should be heard more loudly than theirs when we have more at stake.[64]

When science selects one narrative over another, it is no longer simply involved in an objective production of data. Instead it has assigned a value to those data that places research paradigms and processes ahead of other forms of knowledge production. It may seem unfair or even unreasonable to juxtapose an origin story or oral recounting of a culture's ancestral history against a scientific methodology designed to determine lineage, migration, and customs. But in a case like Kennewick Man, this is precisely the juxtaposition that emerges. Science is not without the same subjective interpretations that are easily attached to cultural stories. If, for example, Ishiguro's Hailsham clones had neither character nor desire and had been simple containers of matching organs, it might not have been as unethical to use them for transplants. Whether or not their existence was a response to an ethical social desire, theirs were the bodies that fulfilled the human desire accomplished through scientific potential. The location of a culture's origin story might seem less consequential than a body's sacrifice—even if the latter is a fiction. Similarly, archaeology's interest in the retrieval of the Ancient One's DNA may seem less of an ethical breach if it leads only to the displacement of a cultural story. But we have assigned that cultural story a significant standing in terms of the rights and privileges of certain citizens. On the face of it, neither an origin story nor a DNA match should have ethical priority. As noted above, the DNA of Kennewick Man could be "used to challenge aboriginal rights to territory, resources and self-determination." In another situation that associates rights and identity, black Cherokees—descendants of freedmen of the 1800s—cannot use DNA to prove their tribal membership. After the 1988 Indian Gaming Regulatory Act boosted the finances of the Five Civilized Tribes of Oklahoma (Cherokee, Chickasaw, Choctaw, Creek, and Seminole), black Cherokees were expunged from the tribal rolls. In 2000, the Seminoles expelled all black members, and in frustration the descendants of the freedmen turned to the courts, and to Rick Kittles. Their hope was that Kittles's DNA tests would prove their tribal blood and effectively challenge their banishment despite the tribes' policy of relying on a text from the 1800s to determine membership. The black descendants wanted science to trump that text. But the tests revealed high percentages of African and European ancestry. In fact, the lowest percentage of "identity"-matched DNA was Native American: the freedmen had just about as much Native American DNA as blacks who had never been on the tribal rolls. Kittles had to explain that the freedmen's ancestors were "no more Indian than blacks in New York City or Baltimore."[65] Sometimes the tests do not map onto our desires.[66]

Whatever the methodologies and outcomes, our blood ties are revived in this urge to use DNA knowledge for individualized medical care—and the ties' vitality is stoked by interests as different as a private wish to locate a personal place of origin and the long-term medical objectives of genomic science. A host of ethically challenging issues lies between that private desire and public utility. The inconsistency of when DNA will count and when it will not is just one of these. DNA evidence has certainly led to ethical and just outcomes, and it has righted injustices, freeing men from prison who had been wrongly convicted of crimes. In these cases, DNA is seen as definitive—but too often recreational DNA assumptions are made about lineage and family that have little scientific reliability.

One DNA-ancestry advocate, Reverend Al Sampson of Chicago, took the paperwork he had received from Kittles's company, African Ancestry, to Lunsar in Sierra Leone.[67] He presented the paperwork to tribal elders, saying: "Five hundred years ago my DNA was removed from here by slave traders and taken to America, so I'm coming back for my seat . . . My seat's been vacant."[68] His story is a fascinating revelation of the social presumptions that are tied to this genetic test. Noting that his DNA (genes, rather than a person) had been taken, he returns to the Sierra Leone to claim his "seat." In what some would see as a very Western claim to property that extends from blood entitlement, Sampson had no difficulty making an association from that test to a legacy, and a "seat." But the DNA test's fragile accuracy regarding ancestral lineages is also clear. How available for private interpretation are identity-based DNA searches? Sampson has started a DNA-based ministry for his congregation. How do these private judgments, perspectives, and ways of looking at the world leak into and impact the public circulation of this technology? The troubling outcomes of recent forays into race-based pharmaceuticals might offer some clues.

The same science that indicates one of its transfers to public knowledge will be pharmaceuticals engineered for genetic individuality has produced pharmaceuticals that are marketed based on race. Although research communities consider these a step toward individualized medicine, how significant is it that we have not been able to get to that individualized endpoint without this aggregate racialized presentation? And how do twenty-first-century populations that have multiracial backgrounds map onto traditional categories of race? This contemporary question cannot be asked outside of the racialized history of medicine. The production of racially targeted pharmaceuticals intersects with this history, which includes the Tuskegee syphilis study mentioned in chapter 1 and discussed in greater detail in chapter 3. The resilient and important Tuskegee narrative has displaced other incidents—both earlier and later—that reveal the persistence and often horror attached to the joint history of race and medicine.[69] The Tuskegee event has taken on a narrative vitality that is sometimes detached from the actual clinical trial. The weaving of narratives around Tuskegee and the way in which we have chosen to tell and remember this story in bioethics is significant in an era when race-based pharmaceuticals often elide or misrepresent that history.

For example, the biopharmaceutical company VaxGen had to abandon plans for its vaccine called AIDSVAX—that preliminary studies suggested would be efficacious for use by black and Asian patients. Criticism of the preliminary data pointed to the shifting ethnic identities that purportedly indicated statistically significant findings.[70] Before the company received FDA approval, the subgroups it thought it had identified as benefiting from the drug were identified as "statistical artifacts," and the drug was withdrawn. In the company's explanation of what had gone wrong with the trial (a statement that had to acknowledge that AIDSVAX had proved ineffective with all trial participants, regardless of race or ethnicity) VaxGen oddly pointed to Tuskegee as the source of its problem, noting that African Americans historically do not participate in clinical trials because of the lingering history of Tuskegee. This reference does not acknowledge that VaxGen had difficulty in general with recruitment for the AIDSVAX trial. The company's reference to Tuskegee as a defense for that difficulty points to its expediency as a public excuse that glosses over a normal expectation of accuracy.[71]

The AIDSVAX debacle was followed by another pharmaceutical company's difficulties marketing BiDil as a drug for African Americans with congestive heart failure. NitroMed's BiDil was the first drug to receive FDA approval for exclusive use by self-identified African Americans. Although the product was announced with great fanfare, sales of the drug fell, and NitroMed's targeted marketing of it had to be abandoned, when evidence emerged that the clinical trials had involved only self-identified African Americans, and that no studies of control groups had been conducted.[72] Another pharmaceutical company, Amgen, has had a similarly difficult time marketing Epogen to patients who, as a result of kidney dialysis, have been disproportionately affected by anemia. Epogen is designed to treat this secondary effect of kidney failure. When charges that Epogen patients had a greater risk of heart attack and death were investigated by the FDA, Amgen asked the Congressional Black Caucus to intervene. The company's argument was that African American patients did not respond well to lower dosages of Epogen, and to deprive them of the drug would be a civil rights injury to black kidney dialysis patients.[73]

Racialized pharmaceutical efforts are likely to have a significant impact on law, politics, and public policy. As the odd reaching out of a pharmaceutical company to the political union of the Congressional Black Caucus indicates, the web of race, science, and society still exists. Just as we cannot separate sordid histories of racial practice and judgment from recreational DNA tests for racial ancestry or from the goal of individualized medicine, we cannot separate the desire for commercial success from pharmaceutical research. Although interests in ancestry are certainly private enterprises that are engaged in by private persons, privacy in the process is not ensured, and the use of the resulting data has not been subjected to the kind of review that should identify and consider the complex ethical issues that accompany the public and private uses of DNA. But that may not be the most troubling aspect of these genomics-based inquiries. Even worse might be the fact that the public use of scientific knowledge works to revive racial categories without interrogating their history. Without a consistent and open review of this potential, and with our national difficulties in substantive engagement with matters of race and gender that point toward social biases, these issues have a potentially deleterious effect on contemporary judgments and evolving genomics-based narratives about race, origin, and difference.

Kazuo Ishiguro understands the consequence of urgency—of questions hurried through review processes so that a result could be accomplished. Years after her Hailsham days, Ishiguro's fictive Kathy meets one of her guardians from the school who urges her to:

> try and see it historically. After the war, in the early fifties, when the great breakthroughs in science followed one after the other so rapidly, there wasn't time to take stock, to ask the sensible questions. Suddenly there were all these new possibilities laid before us, all these ways to cure so many previously incurable conditions. This was what the world noticed the most, wanted the most. And for a long time, people preferred to believe these organs appeared from nowhere, or at most that they grew in a kind of vacuum. Yes, there *were* arguments. But by the time people became concerned . . . there was no way to reverse the process. How can you ask a world that has come to regard cancer as curable, how can you ask such a world to put away that cure, to go back to the dark days? There was no going back.[74]

Ethical inquiry has no certain specified location on the HGP map. No particular path is sketched; there are no indications of where there are mountains or valleys. The allure of a human genome's landscape—the new frontier that was imagined by President Clinton and that recalled the maps of an earlier America—has its own set of symbolic accompaniments: discovery and conquest, horizon and destiny.

It may be left to a fiction that urges our caution. But it is nonetheless a fact that the privacies already threatened in this moment of innovation are difficult to recapture. President Clinton appropriately said that "as we unlock the secrets of the human genome, we must work simultaneously to ensure that new discoveries never pry open the doors of privacy. And we must guarantee that genetic information cannot be used to stigmatize or discriminate against any individual or group."[75]

In the short time that has passed since that announcement, we have already moved to a corporate call for complete disclosure of all genetic information because it is so difficult to maintain privacy in this era of Internet technology.[76] The histories in our words may not be evident in everyday use, but they are nonetheless embedded in our perceptions— even as we try to escape them, and even as we shift our notions of privacy's value or its overestimation. It is absolutely appropriate to notice the ways in which the boundaries and margins of our maps shift, and to be concerned with what motivates the changes of fault lines, and what is recalculated as a result. "There was a certain climate," Ishiguro writes toward the end of *Never Let Me Go,* "and now it's gone."[77]

THREE

Who's Got the Body?

This chapter focuses on clinical trials in medical research and analyzes their impact on "vulnerable" subjects—those whom bioethics considers to be especially at risk with regard to biomedical research. How do those whom bioethicists label as "vulnerable" map onto the identities—women and racial minorities—that are the focus of this book? The history and identity of vulnerable subjects, as well as their exposures in medical trials and the consequences of those trials for them, are the center of this chapter's discussions. Privacy is the value that continues to give a particular contour to the analyses; but in this chapter, the question of privacy is complicated by the questions of maturity (competence), surrogacy, bias, and surveillance that come into play when "vulnerable" populations are the focus, and when these subjects are asked to give their consent to participate in a clinical trial.

• • •

Speaker's Meaning is an extraordinary book by the linguist, philosopher, and barrister Owen Barfield, who wrote about the English language with special attention to how the habits in our use of words reflect both expansions and contractions of meanings. The idea of the book is that a speaker's use of a word is expansive. Contracted meanings, Barfield suggested, are found in lexical (textual) word use. This is a useful dichotomy to keep in mind, especially as we consider some of the lexicon—the words—of ethics and medicine. Consider words as simple as "research," "experiment," and "trial." Then consider the shifts in meanings when these words are paired with "medical" or "clinical": "medical research," "medical experiment," and "clinical trial."

"Clinical trial" is a phrase that came into wide use in the twentieth century. It has emerged as part of the specialist language—for both lexical and spoken texts—that is used to describe a now heavily regulated and highly competitive research industry. In contemporary cultural contexts, "clinical trial" might be considered as an ameliorating phrase, one that bridges the gap between lexical and spoken language. In fact, it has come to occupy the historical place of phrases like "medical experiment." The cultural histories attached to "medical experiment" include the ethical vacuums that were exposed once some of those experiments became public.

The kind of research conducted in a clinical trial may have therapeutic as well as nontherapeutic objectives. If the trial's objective is the choice of one therapy (treatment) over another, the research is therapeutic. For example, in the E-Z measles vaccine trial discussed later in this chapter, the question researchers wanted to answer was which of several drug therapies would be the most efficacious in preventing the disease. If the research is designed to determine more information about a particular disease or disability, but will not have a direct effect on the population enrolled in the trial, even if this population has the disease, the research has nontherapeutic objectives.[1]

A speaker's use of these words can express Barfield's sense of expansion. The words carry memories of social histories. On the other hand, the lexical habits of these words are stripped of these complexities, as the written words focus on particular textual meanings. When we encounter these words in texts about medical research or clinical trials, we are expected to discern their particular intent from the context of their use. This means that we anticipate that the language of medical research will transfer foundational ethical paradigms based on traditional bioethical principles. However, when the actual practices of research betray these codes of conduct, it becomes a moment for social notice. One way this notice is signaled is when speakers use the phrase "medical experiment." It may be a signal that some foundational boundaries have been violated.

There are social and historical reasons why "medical experiment" is not the professional lexicon of choice but appears in spoken vocabulary. That selective use is an effect of "deep structure"—what linguists call the underlying contexts that are merely signaled by the "surface structure," or the spoken word. When speakers of English use the word "experiments," the social histories that can be recalled from the deep structures of use can be haunting and deeply troubling. The spoken word might recall the revelations during the Nuremberg trials of Nazi Germany's heinous experiments on prisoners during the Second World War.[2] Those trials led to the development of professional guidelines for biomedical research that are called the Nuremberg Code, a set of ethical guidelines that are now considered foundational for medical research. As informed consent is the most fundamental ethical standard in biomedical ethics, it is no accident that the first principle in the Nuremberg Code is consent. The first principle in its entirety reads:

> The voluntary *consent* of the human subject is absolutely *essential*. This means that the person involved should have *legal* capacity to give consent; should be so situated as to be able to exercise free power of choice, without the intervention of any element of force, fraud, deceit, duress, over-reaching, or other ulterior form of constraint or coercion; and should have sufficient knowledge and comprehension of the elements of the subject matter involved as to enable him to make an understanding and enlightened decision. This latter element requires that before the acceptance of an affirmative decision by the experimental subject there should be made known to him the nature, duration, and purpose of the experiment; the method and means by which it is to be conducted; all inconveniences and hazards reasonable to be expected; and the effects upon his health or person which may possibly come from his participation in the experiment.[3] [emphasis added]

In the United States, the history of experimentation is attached to populations that ethicists have determined are especially "vulnerable" to medical improprieties. These improprieties are often represented in the literature by what has become a standard reference to the "Tuskegee Study of Untreated Syphilis in the Negro Male"—a now-infamous research experiment that selected 439 African American men in Macon County, Alabama, as research subjects. One hundred and eighty-five men did not have the disease and became the control group. The other 254 men had been diagnosed with syphilis. In order to identify presumed racial distinctions in the manifestations of syphilitic heart disease (which could be determined only during an autopsy), researchers funded by the U.S. Public Health Service did not offer these syphilitic men the standard of care that was readily available to treat (and cure) their disease; failed to elicit their informed consent, contrary to common practices of the time; failed to inform them of the risks of their disease; and unethically offered them incentives to participate in the trial, with the promise of free medical care, transportation, and meals while at the clinic and (for their survivors) burial insurance to assure a quality funeral—a matter that had considerable cultural importance.[4]

The Tuskegee study is just one of a number of experiments conducted in the United States that have not stayed within the normative boundaries of the principled application of medical ethics. Other studies are less commonly cited despite their own circumstances. For example, in the 1920s the social consequence of the scientific embrace of eugenics led to determinations about the value of some citizens over others and forced the sterilizations of women whose procreation was deemed undesirable. State-ordered sterilization was a practice that continued well into the second half of the twentieth century. Many of these sterilizations were attached to determinations that extended the state's interests to the regulation of fertility among certain kinds of women—both white and black, poor, determined to be mentally incompetent, or simply ill (for example, epilepsy was then considered a version of feeblemindedness). One court case in Virginia concerned a seventeen-year-old girl from Charlottesville, Carrie Buck, whom the state determined merited sterilization. The decision to sterilize her was challenged, in part to determine the constitutionality of Virginia's Eugenical Sterilization Act of 1924. The circuit court in Amherst County affirmed the state's right to sterilize Buck, and the U.S. Supreme Court upheld the circuit court's determination.[5] Justice Oliver Wendell Holmes wrote the Court's opinion, which included this now-famous passage: "It is better for all the world, if instead of waiting to execute degenerate offspring for crime or to let them starve for their imbecility, society can prevent those who are manifestly unfit from continuing their kind . . . Three generations of imbeciles are enough."[6]

Chapter 1 reviewed the identitarian constructions of the experiments in birth control carried out within populations that were deemed less desirable by those who supported the hierarchy of eugenics.[7] As late as the last decades of the twentieth century, researchers were able to gain nearly unfettered access to prison populations, children in state institutions, and elderly citizens barely able to give "consent" consistent with the Nuremberg Code.

For example, the Holmesburg Prison Study, in Pennsylvania, has become infamous for its abuses of prisoners.[8] In the fall of 2000, 298 former inmates filed suit against the University of Pennsylvania, Dr. Albert M. Kligman, Johnson and Johnson, and Dow Chemical, charging a wide variety of physical injuries, trauma, and illnesses that resulted from dermatological experiments that included the use of radioactive and carcinogenic materials and hallucinogens, conducted at the prison between 1951 and 1974. The lawsuit alleged that the medical researchers (financed by the pharmaceutical companies named in the lawsuit) exposed prisoners to toxic agents (including dioxin and LSD) without informing them of the potential risks.[9]

The baseline ethical question regarding the Holmesburg case is whether or not men who are incarcerated can be considered autonomous in any way that would allow them to give consent, thus meeting the first standard of clinical trials. When identities such as prisoners, women, or racial and ethnic minorities become coherent enough to be visible, the bioethics question is whether or not these identities emerge because of some medical necessity in the trial (for example, is a prisoner more likely to have a condition related to incarceration?) or whether these identities emerge because of socially constructed biases or social convenience. For medical researchers, the prisoners' location in a single, highly regulated environment made the investigation efficient.

In the early history of this country, the social categorization of enslaved Africans as less than human[10] allowed researchers and physicians to effectively ignore the question of their research subjects' humanity and move forward with experiments or experimental procedures in conditions that would otherwise be seen as inhumane. There is a consistency in the exploited population that extends from the early days of slavery to the end of the twentieth century: the majority of the imprisoned, like the majority of slaves, are African American.[11] This consistency returns us to the matter of identities that are institutionally expedient rather than medically relevant, and that initiate patterns of practice that are difficult to disengage.

DO I CONTRADICT MYSELF?

Recall for a moment the anecdote in the introduction to this book, regarding a question from a physician after my lecture on the subject of identity and privacy. He made an entirely reasonable point concerning my use of the term "body," especially when I was discussing issues of race and gender in bioethics. His quite cogent concern was that in his practice of medicine, he struggled to consider patients as persons, rather than as bodies. His own speaker's preference for "patients" held for him an expansive deep structure that was fully invested with the knowledge that people who came to him for treatment had complex histories and individual experiences. He felt that "body" was a more sterile term— "lexical," in Barfield's vocabulary—and that its use did not encompass the complex individuals who were his patients. In essence, he was describing the difference between a speaker's meaning that expanded, and a lexical meaning that contracted.

A postmodern answer to him—an answer that would allow a wide terrain of complicated and sometimes even competing meanings—would have been that my use of the term "body" functioned for me in the way that "patients" did for him. Sometimes speakers' meanings differ— depending on things like culture, experience, gender, and education. My idea was that "bodies" implied that complexity—and that the word might actually encourage our attentiveness to the complicated and shifting identities that are represented in patient populations.

My use of the word during that lecture and in the chapters of this book encourages some attention to a likely unknowable set of experiences that will not enter directly into the physician's care, but that are still inextricably a part of a person's identity. There is a difference between what a physician learns as the "patient's story" and the unspoken dimensions of that narrative.

One reason to consider fictional narratives is that fiction encourages a reader to tap into a literary imagination that is richer than our personal experiences. Considering an issue from a variety of perspectives is essential for ethicists. Fiction encourages our consideration of perspectives in ways that our personal experiences or the narrowed frames of a case study might not. Fiction also reminds us that despite the absolutely appropriate interests of law, ethics, and medicine in discovering a solution, resolutions are often happenstance and sometimes not very neat. Consider how frequently readers continue thinking past an author's conclusion to a story.

In the past decade, bioethicists have paid substantial attention to "narrative medicine" and the "patient's story."[12] This approach within bioethics acknowledges that the idea of narrative is an unwieldy and wide terrain for the scholars who have embraced this theoretical perspective. Rita Charon explains her use of the term "narrative medicine" to signify the practice of medicine with the "narrative skills of recognizing, absorbing, interpreting, and being moved by the stories of illness." Critical to these skills is the recognition that "narratives of illness . . . grasp patients in all their *complexity*" (emphasis added).[13] Although in my judgment it is an unsuccessful effort, bioethics reaches here toward what Fredric Jameson calls the "ideologeme"—a socially symbolic narrative paradigm that "transforms into texts of a different order."[14] Although contemporary narrative medicine seems to have appeared as a relatively free-standing genre of critique, Jameson's early argument in *The Political Unconscious* explores the politics of social formations from fiction in a way that is related to literary and social disciplines.[15] Perhaps the destination of bioethics' interest is an explanation for its distance from literary theorists' focus on texts. Embracing the complexities of narrative as a vehicle for analysis in medical ethics can seem antithetical to the notion of a focused and resolvable clinical experience. Like law and medicine, bioethics is an investigatory paradigm designed to lead to solutions. Sometimes these cases regard decisions of who should make a "do not resuscitate" order. A surrogate? A patient? The physician? At other times, they involve determining the best standard of care for a premature infant. When narrative ethics is deployed as a vehicle of analysis, we still anticipate that there will be some way of reconciling the instability intrinsic to the idea of narrative that will lead to a stable decision, one that is securely attached to the principles of ethics and that takes into serious consideration the evidence most relevant to the matter under review.

What kind of narrative fiction would be of the most reliable help in this seemingly contradictory task? How can attention to ethics assist our discovery of a viable solution to a medical problem while retaining the open-enedness of narrative? Is there something about the idea of narrative that makes it so capacious that it might even retain some integrity despite its contradictions?

The simple answer to each of these queries is yes. That's what fiction does. The space of the story is already contained by its form. And this form preserves the story even if its elements are contradictory. The nineteenth-century American poet Walt Whitman acknowledged this complexity in the form and content of his classic "Song of Myself." The final lines of the poem are: "Do I contradict myself? / Very well then. I contradict myself. / (I am large. I contain multitudes.)."[16] It is helpful if we recall that the fictional text of the poem is his body. Whitman's expansive idea of his own corporeality expressed here does a wonderful job of illustrating the connection between a person's body and a body of text. But if medical ethics designs paradigms that can assist in the search for a solution or a framework for decision making, how might fictional narratives—which are absolutely open to complex and even contradictory meanings—assist an ethicist in discovering a stable solution to a medical dilemma?

The method of this book's pairing of fact and fiction does not suggest these creative narratives will offer an answer, or even provide a coherent framework that will ultimately be helpful in discovering answers to the ethical questions presented in actual cases. Instead, the practice of using narrative encourages those who recognize that stories are embedded within clinical environments to anticipate that messy habitation and understand that the solution chosen may bear immediate fruit, but may not fully resolve the complications that are implicit in its selection. Whitman, who felt that he, like America, incorporated the very substance of complexity, structurally indicated this inherited terrain in his poem, which celebrated diverse populations that inhabited the new American democracy. His stanzas included expansive lists, illustrating by this example the multitudes that he affirmatively claimed as the contradictions (given his poem's self-referential title) within him and within America:

> The pure contralto / . . . The carpenter / . . . The married and unmarried children / . . . The pilot / . . . The mate / . . . The duck-shooter / . . . The deacons / . . . The spinning-girl / . . . The farmer / . . . The lunatic / . . . The quadroon girl / . . . The machinist / . . . the policeman / . . . the gate-keeper / . . . The half-breed / . . . The squaw / . . . The connoisseur / . . . the deck-hands / . . . The young sister / . . . The one-year wife / . . . The clean-hair'd Yankee girl / . . . The paving-man / . . . the shoemaker / . . . The conductor / . . . The child / . . . The peddler / . . . The bride / . . . The opium-eater / . . . The prostitute / . . . The President / . . . The Missourian / . . . the fare-collector / . . . the tinners / . . . the masons / . . . Patriarchs . . . sons . . . grandsons . . . great-grandsons. . . . And these tend inward to me, and I tend outward to them, / And such as it is to be of these more or less I am, / And of these one and all I weave the song of myself.[17]

A citation of this length illustrates how his poem managed the complexity of his idea by inclusive and repetitive structures. These narratives overcome the implicit contractions of a narrowed textual lexicon with devices that accomplish a speaker's habits of expansion. Whitman's stanza-length lists structure this methodological interest. But making meaning in fiction is different from making meaning in speech. Transcriptions, a medical case, or a patient's history do not automatically become narrative text simply because we read it or because we relate it to poetry or prose. The stories that have become a focus in narrative bioethics were formed as medical speech, and it is important to remember that making meaning from speech includes our willingness to understand its origin. Although bioethics has appropriately evinced much interest in narratology, this is perhaps the most important constraint when narratology encourages our attention to the patient's story. Certainly the narrative judgment in *Buck v. Bell* begged for some attention to the cultural construction of the legal narrative and the medical presumptions that composed it.

Acknowledgment of narrative complexity does not mean that fiction is an unreliable interlocutor. Certainly the construction of meaning is not as simple a matter as opening a book to its first page and reading through to the end. It includes the spaces between, where fiction is intentionally thickened by an author's creative imagination and where tone, settings, subplots, and minor characters express the social and cultural histories of the text. And if all of these were not complicated enough, they are all joined by the reader's critical engagement.

One of the most important lines in *Jazz*, the novel by the American writer Toni Morrison, comes at the end of the book, where the narrative voice reaches out to the reader: "Look. Look where your hands are. Now."[18] If the reader follows that instruction, she will look down to see that she is holding Morrison's book in her hands. Morrison identifies her reader as critical to the narrative act—making meaning. The act of reading brings the story to its telling. The deep structures of vocabulary that come from a reader's experience contribute to all the devices of narrative. The author's text is certainly the provocateur, but reading makes meaning. At the very least, a meeting between lexical and spoken texts extends our own experiential corpus. This convergence is useful to bioethics.

The philosopher Martha Nussbaum comes closest to suggesting what the interdisciplinary collage of cases and texts that contribute the stories in this book might offer a reader when she writes that "moral knowledge ... is perception. It is seeing a complex, concrete reality in a highly lucid and richly responsive way; it is taking in what is there, with imagination and feeling."[19] If you are an ethicist faced with a decision about whether it is right or wrong to implant a half-dozen fertilized eggs in a patient who already has six children,[20] the suggestion to look toward your imagination and discover how you "feel" about the matter is, quite frankly, unsatisfactory. Bioethics' principles (autonomy, beneficence, justice, and nonmaleficence) reflect an effort to capture a common morality and offer a critical framework for these feelings.[21] When we consider the composition of research populations in clinical trials, ethics' interest in neutrality demands that a patient's identity outside of the medical matters that make him or her a reasonable subject for the trial be an irrelevant factor in that person's participation. Of course, identity can matter in clinical trials in a way that is both necessary and appropriate.

The reason that bioethics has become so necessary to the assessment of clinical trials is that contemporary practices in medicine are traceable to the patterns of past conduct, which can compromise the ethical neutrality that should structure these trials. Populations must be appropriately screened. A trial for a uterine cancer drug should involve women. And it would certainly be unreasonable for a trial for a prostate cancer drug to include women. But when should children be an appropriate population for a clinical trial for a drug to combat leukemia? How old should they be, and who should make these decisions?

At the same time that there are reasonable claims to selecting certain identities and excluding others, issues of race, gender, situation, and age are open to the narrative histories of the United States and vulnerable to the biases that have accompanied our social understandings of the rights accorded to women, children, and racial and ethnic minorities. Social histories do not disappear from the extensive deep structures of our judgments, and evidence throughout the twentieth century indicates that our clinical judgment has too often been less than neutral, even though at one point in our history those judgments seemed informed by the latest science—science that included eugenics.

In the history of medicine, populations labeled as "vulnerable" are patients whose medical care has been attached to identity. Remember that there are appropriate medical markers of identity for clinical trials. But in cases where ethics goes missing, it has been social identity, rather than medical judgment, that selects the populations. The ethicists Anna Mastroianni and Jeffrey Kahn trace this history from the moment that the "exploitation of 'vulnerable' subject populations . . . came to light between the mid-1960s and the early 1970s."[22] They recall "landmark examples" (Susan Reverby, including the Tuskegee experiments, refers to these as the "holy trinity" of bioethics)—hepatitis vaccine research on institutionalized children at the Willowbrook State School in New York State[23] and a research protocol that called for "the injection of live cancer cells into elderly nursing home residents" by researchers at the Jewish Chronic Disease Hospital in New York.[24] Mastroianni and Kahn introduce a third experiment in their discussion of justice and human subject research with an adjectival phrase offered without further explanation: the "'so-called' Tuskegee Syphilis Study."[25] In their overview of the evolution of justice in human subjects research, the authors note that each of these studies focused on regulations that were particularly concerned with populations that Mastroianni and Kahn list as groups "namely, prisoners, children, and pregnant women and fetuses" that have subsequently been singled out for additional protections.[26]

However, in a puzzling lacuna, not once are the subjects of the Tuskegee syphilis study ever identified in the text of the essay as black men. Nevertheless, the Tuskegee study is arguably the most readily identifiable as unethical by professional and lay people. Although Mastroianni and Kahn do not state this explicitly, "vulnerable" refers to patients who are exploitable with regard to medical abuses that are attached to the social biases regarding identity. It is important to clarify this definition.

The Tuskegee syphilis study has become the most infamous medical trial in the United States. In spoken language the nearly pejorative word "experiment" is more common than the more innocuous term "study," which appears as the lexical representation of the event.[27] The differences express a judgment about the consequences and processes of the trial, especially the consistently vigorous public misunderstanding regarding the study's procedure—an incorrect belief that the physicians in charge injected the subjects with syphilis. But rather than reexamine this well-rehearsed case, let us use a different focus on the Tuskegee study, examining its representational force in bioethics.[28] What has made it the ur-text in ethics' studies of clinical trials? Even Mastroianni and Kahn's brief reference to it in their list of exemplary studies that forced reconsideration of ethics and human subjects research indicates that it is a primary text.[29]

It could be that the government's involvement in the study that refused treatment to these research subjects when one was readily available for their condition makes it of particular import.[30] It is important to recall that the differences the researchers anticipated would only be discoverable upon autopsy—which led to their offering burial incentives to families if they would allow physicians to perform the autopsy that they anticipated would validate their theory that syphilitic heart disease manifested itself differently in white bodies than in black ones. If we read Tuskegee in this way, our attention shifts from the researchers' ethical malfeasance. Instead the amorphous terrain of the federal government's participation makes a (narratively) more compelling case for assessment and blame. This is a shift in perspective similar to asking what biases physicians might bring to the treatment of minority breast cancer patients that makes these women less likely to receive aggressive care, rather than asking the more commonly posed question: what do minority breast cancer patients fail to do that explains the less aggressive care they receive?[31] Another reason for the displacement of other, similarly offensive violations of ethics in clinical trials in the teaching of ethics could be that the narrative of Tuskegee is so ubiquitous that it needs little more than a nodding reference—"Of course you know about Tuskegee?"—to evoke the complex story.

An alternative argument that might explain why Tuskegee retains its prominence—with the resulting lack of attention to other, equally egregious cases—exposes a difficulty that harkens back to my opening statement that matters of race expose unease in bioethics. This perspective suggests that engaging this story, rehearsing its details, and analyzing its era animates the very biases that created the environment for the "experiment" to last for nearly half a century, despite the knowledge of otherwise esteemed practitioners in the medical and research fields. In other words, the Tuskegee narrative remains preeminent because the idea of black male sexuality, embedded in the narrative of the event as well as in its public notice, has some perverse appeal to the public's consumption of the story. It is not unreasonable to consider that some engagement of the pejorative association between black male sexuality and disease has filtered into the public narrative. This consideration explains the persistence and popularity of narratives that involve sexuality, race, and disease.

The word "clinical" comes from a twentieth-century expansion of the word "clinic." Its lexical use suggests something that is "coldly detached." But when a disease trend is paired with a "vulnerable" population, the narrative loses the anticipated detached status. Patients' backgrounds, gender, social status, and race attach to a speaker's (expansive) discourse and sever the potential for neutrality. For example, researchers could not conduct trials of birth control pills in the continental United States because a set of federal and state statutes prevented the dissemination there of information regarding contraceptives. These laws prevailed until 1965 when the Supreme Court, in *Griswold v. Connecticut*, struck down the remaining statutes.[32] Researchers chose the new district of Rio Piedras in Puerto Rico for the trials. In *Contagious: Cultures, Carriers, and the Outbreak Narrative*, the literature professor Priscilla Wald recalls the outrage that the journalist Jacob Riis experienced while listening to the reports of the New York State Tenement House Commission regarding the conditions of tenements in the mid-1880s. Riis wrote: "The truth [is that] in the tenements all the influences make for evil; because they are the hot-beds of epidemics that carry death to rich and poor alike . . . they touch the family life with deadly moral contagion. This is their worst crime, inseparable from the system."[33] Wald writes that tenements provoked a "particular association of those spaces with immigrants [that] intensified nativism by materializing and amplifying the fear of communicable-disease epidemics imported by immigrants and bred by the squalor of the tenements."[34] Contemporary subsidized public housing is the successor to tenements, with the same lack of protection of the residents' privacy.[35]

It was not difficult to notice the class of "others" who promoted disease, who became "vulnerable" research populations, or who raised stereotypes in the minds of the physicians and other health care workers who came into contact with these patients. These were citizens whose residence rendered them less private or whose appearance connected them to negative social stereotypes. Gender is also a potential other in this mix. It is important to recognize that "gender" does not only signal an interest in women, despite the way in which the term is used in everyday speech. "Gender" also refers to men, as the Tuskegee study indicated. In this book, when gender matters, one sex or the other is significant in the evolution of the medical narrative. In the case of Tuskegee, the social history that recounts a national fear of black male sexuality is at issue.[36] Social biases regarding expressive sexuality accompany the idea of "black male" for many English speakers, and that fact is unlikely to be inconsequential in either the events or the memory of the Tuskegee study.

One important social marker of the boundary between private and public that has become increasingly important is the emergence of "public" health concerns in the United States.[37] Those populations that were the focus of public health fears and thus subject to public health regulations became the "vulnerable" populations that Mastroianni and Kahn included in their essay. Some have been institutionalized by the state (in prisons or hospitals) and subsequently lost their autonomy. Some are urban poor—usually minorities—who cannot afford private health insurance and in this way become subject to state policies regarding the dispensation of medical treatments. These treatments range from reproductive health care, well-baby care, nutrition, mental-health care, and access to medical tests. Some are women; others are men who have some social stereotype attached to them that mitigates against their having fully autonomous personhood in the area of rights.

The differences between vulnerable bodies that become public because of some visible identity and those that can remain private because of a privileged autonomy urges a cultural bioethics to consider the complication of those identities. Privacy is the norm from which identity values vary. As a value that has constitutional and individual saliency, privacy matters. What happens when a patient's body is not invested with the normative protection of the private? One answer to the physician who wondered at my use of the word "body" as opposed to his preferred "patient" might have been that even when a patient's story or background are unknown, a visible identity offers a text that begins to act on what we believe we understand about a body even before any interaction other than vision occurs. Is a body useful, or autonomous?

BROTHERS OR SISTERS?

Is there a point when a reader of Jodi Picoult's novel *My Sister's Keeper* might pause to consider the gendered shift of the biblical adage that the title gestures toward, and that the first pages recall, with Anna's traumatic recollection that "in my first memory I am three years old and trying to kill my sister"?[38] Picoult might have considered that Cain's query to God—"Am I my brother's keeper?"—is so common a text that it needed nothing further than this semantic shift to echo the question posed in the Book of Genesis. The cadence alone prompts a familiarity that might be enough to signal the novel's focus. But Picoult's creative license is evident when she changes essential dimensions of the question and the event—the gender of the sibling, as well as making the question into a statement. For the children in this novel, the title stands as a stark and powerful declaration, the core of a story about two sisters who struggle through a relationship that began when one of them (Kate) developed life-threatening leukemia and the younger (Anna) was conceived and selected—through pre-implantation genetic diagnosis, or PGD—to be a donor for her older sister's increasingly invasive medical needs.

Picoult's novel begins when Anna, who feels as if she "didn't seem to exist, except in relation to her (sister)" seeks a lawyer who will represent her in an effort to emancipate herself from her parents. As she tells the startled attorney, "I want to sue them for the rights to my own body."[39]

Anna and Kate are not alone in this troubled family. The parents are pitiful figures themselves, struggling to fulfill multiple roles: lifesaver for their older daughter, spousal partners, professionals (she is a lawyer, he is a firefighter), and parents to their two other children, Anna and Jesse. Their son's hidden needs threaten the fragile family bonds nearly as seriously as Anna's lawsuit. Jesse sets secret fires and enjoys the havoc they create and the excitement they produce in the firefighters (including his father) who must respond to them. But like his father, he is a subtext, a nearly silent participant in the story that focuses on his two sisters,[40] who struggle with the matter of genetic matching that renders one of them a donor—and an increasingly necessary one—for the other.

The mother is the most visible parent in the story, and in this regard, the narrative is a gendered one: the triad of the mother and her daughters controls the evolution of the ethical conundrums in this story, whose most prominent question is whether one sister should be able to legally emancipate herself from her parents and call a halt to the use of her body as medical salvage for her sister.

The family's attentions are brutally divided. The parents, Brian and Sara Fitzgerald, see themselves as "a pair of sentries, a double line of defense" against the omnipresent potential of death.[41] For fifteen years they have managed to keep their terminally ill daughter alive. But then the enemy shifts from the disease of the older girl to their thirteen-year-old daughter, who informs them (through her lawyer) that she wants to stop the increasingly invasive and painful tests and procedures. The consequence of her decision is that Kate will die without the donation of Anna's cellular material.

Consider the deep structure in the idea of donation. As text, the word has a restricted meaning that relates it to a gift. Even though Sara is speaking in Picoult's text, the textual representation suggests the restricted idea of donation, as shown in this sample of a remark from Sara: "When we had Anna, I remind Brian, we knew she was going to be a donor for Kate."[42] Of course, the central ethical question is whether or not Anna can be an altruistic donor at all. Aren't her actions compelled by her parents' implicit powers of substituted judgment?[43]

Picoult writes effectively of how stunned the parents are to discover that Anna has expressed any individual, autonomous desire at all, and that her desire might be legally viable. The descriptive literary language assists the story's slow, but nonetheless incendiary, development. The narrative is sprinkled with fiery images like "ax" and "ignites." And the ethical landscape is deeply engaging in this story that focuses on family and individuality—and especially the "right" to one's "own body." Brian, the father, says to his wife:

"I think we need to give Anna a chance to explain. We *agreed* to give her a chance to explain, right?"

I duck my head. "I don't want to do it anymore."

That ignites my mother. "Well, you know Anna, neither do I. In fact, neither does Kate. But it's not something we have a choice about."

The thing is, I *do* have a choice. Which is exactly why I have to be the one to do this . . .

"For God's sake, Anna," my mother says. "Do you even realize what the consequences would be?"[44]

Is there a point in the story where it is significant to the narrative that the brother is sidelined and one sister is posed as the keeper of the other? Picoult's decision to make subtle shifts in narrative emphasis and our notice of them (or not) reflect the ethical terrain that the choices we make about women and girls and about boys occupy. Picoult seems to have assumed that her readers would be content to have the brother's troubles remain a subtext, until he becomes so dangerous a pyromaniac that his actions (in some ways, not dissimilar to those of Anna) threaten the fragile moral and structural coherence of the family.

Picoult describes one of these fires with references that reach to the troubled household that contains her story: "In a burning house, your sixth sense kicks in. You can't see, because of the smoke. You can't hear, because fire roars loud. You can't touch, because it will be the end of you."[45]

When the Fitzgeralds' own home is figuratively a house afire, the reader is in a position to provide an ethical balance—a form of sixth sense. In the novel, the law attempts this role. Not only does it step into the fray when the court appoints a guardian ad litem for Anna, but it is also the alternative to the medical narrative that has no solution to the crises of a donor who refuses to part with the "gift" of her body.

One way to read the conundrums of medical ethics that are at the novel's center, and to consider their impact, is to begin with the ethical questions that are embedded in the decision of the parents to undergo selective reduction of the fertilized eggs to select the one most likely to be compatible with their terminally ill daughter. They attempt to address the ethical questions of the event when challenged by reporters who get wind of the story and challenge their moral judgment. They respond: "We didn't ask for a baby with blue eyes, or one that would grow to be six feet tall, or one that would have an IQ of two hundred. Sure we asked for specific characteristics—but they're not anything anyone would ever consider to be model human traits. They're just *Kate's* traits. We don't want a superbaby. We just want to save our daughter's life."[46]

Their clarification here is effectively an admission that their interest in Kate goes beyond the range of their ethical inquiry. Did they have an obligation in their decision making to consider the autonomy of the other child, and the appropriate domains of parental surrogacy? Should there have been some consideration for the ethical autonomy of the child birthed for her biological usefulness to her sister?

A case that resonates with the exchange of sibling body parts occurred at Columbia University's Lowenstein Center for the Study and Prevention of Childhood Disruptive Behavior Disorders and the New York State Psychiatric Institute, in New York City. At least thirty-four boys, between the ages of seven and eleven, became participants in a study that hypothesized a link between violence and genetics. The boys were "44 percent black and 56 percent Hispanic."[47] Harriet Washington cites the observation of Ruby Brown, the lawyer for Charisse Johnson, who brought suit against the two institutions, alleging that "all the 'Hispanic' boys lived in the Washington Heights area and were black Dominicans."[48]

The research project was led by Daniel Pine and Gail Wasserman of Columbia University, who studied the younger male siblings of "male offenders in an effort to identify early predictors of antisocial behavior." The subjects were referred to researchers by the probation department, despite the supposed privacy of juvenile records.[49]

The boys were doubly vulnerable. They were ethnic and/or racial minorities, and their older brothers were involved with the probation department—specifically, the subjects were the younger brothers of convicted delinquents. With sentiments that are reminiscent of those of parents who signed consent forms for their children to be injected with the hepatitis vaccine at Willowbrook, one of the boys' parents noted: "I felt at the time that if they could find me and knew I had a six year old son they had enough power to affect the wellbeing of my sixteen year old son who was being held in a detention facility."[50] In contract law, these are called contracts of adhesion—agreements that are imbalanced. Leonard Glantz summarizes the process:

> The investigators then visited the children's homes to rate them on a number of variables. Finally, the investigators assessed the boys' sero-tonergic activity based on prior work that supposedly shows a relationship between serotonin levels and aggression. To accomplish this, all boys were free of medications for at least one month, all followed a low-monoamine diet for four days, and all fasted the night before the test (referred to as a "challenge"). On the day of the challenge, the boys received nothing by mouth and an intravenous catheter was inserted at 8:30 A.M. and remained in place for about five and a half hours. Researchers orally administered fenfluramine hydrochloride to the boys at 10:00 A.M. and took blood samples every hour from the catheter. By measuring certain biochemical responses to the fen-fluramine challenge, the investigators would be able to make an assessment of the boys' central serotonergic activity. The investigators conducted this research in an attempt "to replicate results that have suggested that aggression in prepubertal children is positively correlated with central serotonergic activity" and to determine if "an association between adverse-rearing conditions and serotonin in children" existed.[51]

The ethical questions that emerge from this study are multifaceted. In addition to noting that researchers continued the protocol and did not release children who complained of headaches or lightheadedness, it is important to note that fenfluramine was the drug (under the name Fen-Phen) that the FDA banned in 1997 because of its associations with heart valve damage and death.[52] But the issues of privacy and autonomy also loom large. These children, like Anna, became of medical interest because of their siblings. What say did they have in their enrollment in this trial? What psychological impact is there when a youngster becomes visible because of a brother's or sister's legal or medical situation? What is a child's reasonable claim to privacy? Is what happens in a home—even if it is a form of clinical trial—a private matter?

MINI-CLINICAL TRIALS

Anna's desire for her parents to appreciate her own personhood is frustrated by another role the parents claim for themselves—the managers of what is effectively a family-centered, medically authorized mini-clinical trial. One physician researcher reminded me that "parents practice 'mini-clinical trials' on their children all the time."[53] Although she was referring to parents who "experiment" with different over-the-counter cough medicines to see which one is more effective, the particular issues that attach to children's autonomy and medical profiles eventually led to a 2008 regulation that required that new drugs and new formulations of existing drugs undergo clinical trials before being prescribed for children.[54] Clinical trials that happen in the privacy of the home can end up in the courtroom. Consider, for example, cases that mix issues of religious freedom and illness, as when a parent tries to cure a child's illness through prayer in the privacy of their home, or seeks out nontraditional treatments for an ill child. Is there a private right to determine the care (and the origin of that care) for your child?

Something about the nature of privacy now constitutionally attached to pregnant women has seeped into the widening landscape of IVF and other reproductive technologies. The idea of the fetus itself and maternal privacy, addressed in *Roe v. Wade*, has a much wider narrative terrain than that imagined in the 1973 Supreme Court decision. And when these privately practiced technologies reach the public sphere, Picoult's fiction is not too different from real events.

A survey from the Johns Hopkins University's Genetics and Public Policy Center indicated that 61 percent of Americans supported the selection of a "savior sibling" through genetic testing of embryos.[55] But the support for the use of this technology within the survey's respondents disappeared when other factors were introduced—such as sex selection.

In the 1980s Mary and Abraham Ayala were faced with the certain death of their daughter Anissa, from chronic myelogenous leukemia. They had another daughter, Marissa—in the hope that she would be a match for her sixteen-year-old sister. When their younger daughter was just over a year old, she donated bone marrow for her sister's use, a process that included anesthetizing and hospitalizing Marissa. The germ of Picoult's novel may have come from the controversy that surrounded this case, but there were subsequent cases as well. For instance, in 1999 Lisa and Jack Nash used PGD to attempt to have another child who could be a donor for their daughter, Molly, who had Fanconi's anemia (a son was born in 2000, and was a match for his sister). The Nash family was British, but because England's Human Fertilisation and Embryology Authority declined permission for PGD for a family whose son had Diamond-Blackfan anemia, the Nashes traveled to the United States to undergo PGD hoping they could give birth to a child who would be a donor for their daughter.

There are certainly good reasons to except these cases from a standard understanding of clinical trials. Yet they do raise profound ethical questions that cause some survey respondents to accept the idea of a family's having a "savior baby" but refuse to endorse what is popularly called the "designer baby"—a child planned just as intentionally as a "savior baby," but not conceived for the purpose of keeping another person alive. Picoult's novel captures the public concern over these private practices and the ways in which reproductive choices for women—despite the father's necessary contribution of sperm—carry the narrative weight of the event. In the late 1980s, the Ayalas had only a one in four chance that their new baby would be a match for their teenaged daughter. Was either their pregnancy or the use of the younger daughter's bone marrow a matter of experimentation? Or must a clinical trial only involve a larger population, the standard controls of scientific experiments, oversight by an institutional review board (IRB), and the various other mechanisms that have been deployed to make certain that events like Tuskegee and Willowbrook do not happen again in U.S. medicine?[56]

One way to consider the similarities and differences here is to identify the ethical concerns and see if they connect to particular populations. In other words, how does identity matter in an ethical review?

If the question is asked this way, children certainly seem to have a particular vulnerability that would cause a reasonable person—and this is the standard used in the law—to hesitate before determining that their participation in a medical trial needs no particular oversight. Mastroianni and Kahn include children as vulnerable populations, along with the institutionalized and the elderly.[57] The history of experimentation on those who are in vulnerable social positions arguably merits the same caution, and a similar hesitation. This is why it is difficult to separate the social context from the medical, despite the sometimes selective interest in bioethics in doing precisely that.

A SITUATIONAL BIOETHICS?

J. Marion Sims, known as the father of modern gynecology, was unhappy to discover that the operation he had perfected after practicing on enslaved women who suffered from vesicovaginal fistulas was not earning him the attention he felt it should. In fact, in his 1884 autobiography, Sims complained about his situation:

> Other doctors were performing all these operations very successfully in the other hospitals. I could not advertise; I could get nothing to do; I had no means of bringing myself before the public or of reaching the profession, because I had no hospital in which to operate or to perform these marvelous operations. As soon as the doctors had learned what they wanted of me, they dropped me . . . My thunder had been stolen, and I was left without any resources whatever. I said to myself, "I am a lost man unless I can get somebody to create a place in which I can show the world what I am capable of doing."[58]

Sims did not record the use of anesthetics during his surgeries on slave women even though later, in his autobiography, he wrote: "In America, accoucheurs use chloroform and surgeons mostly use ether. I believe there has not as yet been a single death from chloroform administered during labor."[59] But he cautions about the use of chloroform rather than ether in "surgical operations," noting that "ether . . . is safe in purely surgical cases."[60] It does not seem inappropriate, given Sims's commentary, to question his failure to use palliative drugs during his surgeries on enslaved women to relieve the extraordinarily painful conditions produced by their fistulas and the pain of the surgical procedures they endured. But as indicated in chapter 1, there is no consensus of opinion here. What is the appropriate place for history when we judge the ethics of past events? Does identity have a role in producing the tone of any of this debate? Lewis Wall, an M.D. who is known for fistula surgeries in Ethiopia, embraces one extreme: "There is no doubt that slaves in the mid-19th century American South were a 'vulnerable' population who were often subjected to significant abuse by the slaveholding system. To suggest, however, that for that reason alone no attempts should have been made to cure the maladies of such enslaved women, especially when they were desperate for help and no other viable alternatives existed, seems ethically bankrupt itself."[61]

Is the ethical argument indeed reducible to a choice between no operation at all and an operation without the assistance of anesthetics that were routinely provided to women in labor at that time?

My comment in the introduction about the difficulty medical ethics has in engaging with racial issues seems particularly relevant to Sims's experiments and to the Tuskegee study. But what happens when race is removed from the equation and women are the focus of clinical trials? Picoult's novel effectively erases the husband and son from the major plot, leaving the drama to develop between the mother and her daughters. Does this gendered emphasis have an effect on the narrative's dramatic potential? How?

It is difficult to remove visible identities from these scenarios. The birth control trials in Puerto Rico indicated that ethnicity has indeed produced differences in trial protocols and in experimental drug levels. Sue Rosser, a professor of history, technology, and society, explores the ways in which "women of color have become the target for particular aspects of women's health research," noting that "often these areas represent issues of social concern or social problems." She cites research that focuses on black teenage pregnancy and a spate of studies during the 1990s that were designed to assess the "prevalence of substance abuse during pregnancy" that studied frequencies in inner-urban hospitals only "where the substance-abuse frequency was found to be higher [among] women of color"—research that helped "to establish the baseline data which have led to laws" mandating that physicians report women who are suspected of using drugs or alcohol during their pregnancy.[62] Of course, the issues of privacy and confidentiality are absolutely relevant to a consideration of physicians' reporting patients' drug use. Which drugs? And what populations? Is this a warrantless search, of the kind that is constitutionally impermissible? The legal scholar Dorothy Roberts reviewed an article about women who received prenatal care in public health offices or in private obstetrical offices in Pinellas County, Florida.[63] Roberts interprets the result, noting that even though "there was little difference in the prevalence of substance abuse by pregnant women along either racial or economic lines, nor was there any significant difference found between public clinics and private offices . . . Black women were ten times more likely than whites to be reported to government authorities. Both public health facilities and private doctors were more inclined to turn in Black women than white women for using drugs while pregnant."[64]

Roberts's example illustrates the bodies at stake in Rosser's book. But in a discussion of how identity might matter in clinical trials, it is important to recall another point made by Rosser: that when women of color are included in medical research they "too often become misused as subjects in experiments which either lend credence to racial stereotypes or fail to distinguish true health problems among women."[65]

The World Medical Assembly's "Declaration of Helsinki: Ethical Principles for Research Involving Human Subjects" reflects agreements that date back to 1964. The primary audiences for Helsinki declarations like this are physicians and researchers. Yet, given the abuses that still emerge in human subject research, it is reasonable to ask whether or not the Helsinki declarations have led to exemplary conduct when experimenting with human subjects.[66] If this is not the case, why not—especially given the extraordinary levels of regulatory oversight from institutional review boards, hospital ethics committees, and academic and corporate attention to research on human subjects?

In 1998 the NIH investigated a study in Los Angeles that was designed to determine whether a vaccine—the Edmonston-Zagreb, or E-Z, measles vaccine—could be given to infants only four months old. Medical researchers at the Johns Hopkins University and the Centers for Disease Control and Prevention (CDC) cooperated in the study, which distributed the vaccine in Haiti, Peru, Thailand, Uzbekistan, and the African countries of Cameroon, Egypt, Gambia, Rwanda, South Africa, the Sudan, Togo, and Zaire. Haitian infants were administered doses at ten to five hundred times the usual levels. The trials in the United States vaccinated children from Los Angeles. These populations were, like the global populations of the study, overwhelmingly urban-dwelling, black or brown minority children. The study began during a measles epidemic in the United States and, according to the *Los Angeles Times*, it "was conducted on nearly 1,500 minority infants in Los Angeles [and it] failed to disclose to parents that one of the vaccines was experimental." The studies were defended by David Satcher, who was the director of the CDC during the time of the trial. He later became surgeon general. In commenting on that fact that Kaiser Permanente of California, which distributed the drug to babies in Los Angeles, had failed to inform parents that their children were receiving an experimental dose of the vaccine, Satcher called it a "little mistake."[67] The *Los Angeles Times* article noted:

> The informed consent papers signed by parents, which were reviewed and approved by institutional review boards at the CDC and Kaiser, said children would receive one of two vaccines and that two different doses of the E-Z vaccine would be studied. The form did not say that E-Z was experimental or unlicensed . . . Researchers became concerned in 1990 and 1991 when data from studies in Senegal and Guinea-Bissau, and later from Haiti, suggested an increased death rate among female infants receiving the stronger dose of the E-Z vaccine.[68]

News reports, although informative, should not be the final source of information about this study. One could reasonably anticipate that the E-Z measles trials would receive as vigorous a review in the bioethics community as Tuskegee had. Certainly the public narratives placed the event in the context of bias rather than in the category of more neutral clinical trials that may commit errors of judgment, but those narratives of bias still seem idiosyncratic rather than falling into a predictable pattern of flawed medical experimentation.

Questions regarding how race and age factored into the study would reasonably seem to be of particular concern to medical researchers who are understandably anxious not to repeat either the history or the pattern of Tuskegee in dealing with vulnerable communities. Nevertheless, it is critical to this analysis to understand the population demographic. Unless the text is race and ethics, it is difficult to find commentary on and analyses of the ethical flaws in the measles vaccine trials in contemporary ethics literature.[69]

My Sister's Keeper warns its readers about issues concerning identity that—because of adult desires or urgency, or some hierarchy of social or cultural needs—may become noticeable only in a crisis, as when Anna asks for liberation from her parents, or a reporter exposes cases like Tuskegee or the E-Z vaccine trials.

Picoult's novel insists that the reader recognize the complex and sometimes contradictory impulses of children. There are no easy ways to create protocols for the messy constitutions of families, neighborhoods, or communities in clinical trials. But perhaps regulatory protocols are not the only way to direct our attention to those who—because of age, status, or other dimensions of identity—become subjects in a clinical trial.

CONSENT, CONSULTATION, AND COMMUNITIES

As noted earlier, informed consent is the most basic ethical standard in clinical trials. This is the principle that is immediately at issue when the parents in Picoult's novel use their new daughter's stem cord blood to treat their child with leukemia. To whom did the stem cord blood belong? The baby or the mother? This might be the least complicated ethical question in the novel because the umbilical cord is detached from both mother and child; but its use nonetheless begins the path down a slippery slope of procedures that do unquestionably violate the autonomy of the "donor," become invasive, cause pain and psychological damage, and otherwise compromise her standard of life. Even "donor" in this novel is a questionable category. The word implies an altruistic gift, but because Anna was a minor, her "gifts" to her sister were determined by her legally authorized surrogates—her parents—whose compromised objectivity determines the course of events in the story.

But what of adults whose informed consent is waived? What situations might render their private authority—their autonomy—over their own bodies moot in the way that Anna finally finds unacceptable, as Kate becomes increasingly dependent on her biological material?

Ruth Faden and Tom Beauchamp provide a thoughtful analysis of the concept of informed consent, noting that "informed consent is analyzable in terms of the web of cultural and policy rules and requirements of consent that collectively form the social practice of informed consent in instructional contexts where *groups* of patients and subjects must be treated in accordance with rules, policies, and standard practices. Here, informed consents are not always *autonomous* acts, nor are they always in any meaningful respect *authorizations*."[70]

Faden and Beauchamp argue that informed consent is synonymous with an "autonomous authorization"[71] and that whatever name we give it, this action yields substantial authority to someone else. Subjects in a clinical trial do not devise and administer a cocktail of drugs that might or might not be effective in the treatment of HIV/AIDS, but they authorize someone else to do so.[72] Considering the critical role that "authorization" and "authority" play in the process of informed consent, Faden and Beauchamp whittle down this definition with a determination that "an informed consent . . . is given if a patient or subject with (1) substantial understanding and (2) in substantial absence of control by others (3) intentionally (4) authorizes a professional" to act.[73]

If we apply this definition to Picoult's novel, it makes it relatively simple to name what it was that Anna lacked, and what authority her parents claimed. But advances in medicine are not always made within such clearly articulated (if not necessarily defensible) contexts. The providers of emergency medicine, for example, have requested that this authority be removed from patients who are in life-threatening situations and whose traumatic injuries make it impossible for them to give consent.

One example of a clinical trial that proceeded with the waiver of informed consent from participants was the trial of an artificial blood substitute, PolyHeme, produced by Northfield Laboratories. The company requested the waiver under the aegis of an amended FDA regulation that included "emergency research" in guidelines for Exception from Informed Consent (EFIC) for research in emergency medicine when "the human subjects are in life-threatening situations . . . and the collection of randomized placebo controlled investigations is necessary to determine the safety and effectiveness of particular interventions."[74] The matter of informed consent becomes even more complicated when consent is compromised. Are some bodies more likely than others to become research subjects when informed consent is waived under EFIC guidelines? Are their populations vulnerable to particular demographics?

PolyHeme's patient population was a randomly selected group of men and women whom emergency medical technicians (EMTs) were transporting to an emergency room and who had lost substantial quantities of blood—so much so that a transfusion was indicated. Because EMTs do not carry whole blood, the PolyHeme trial was designed to see whether an artificially manufactured blood product would be better than (or as good as) saline delivered en route to the hospital. The trial was randomized so that some ambulance patients received saline followed by the regular protocol of typing and then transfusing whole blood in the hospital. But during the in-house phase of the trial those ambulance patients who got PolyHeme in transit continued to receive the artificial product for at least twelve hours after admission to the hospital. Some bioethicists—including those at Massachusetts General Hospital who refused to take part in the trial—found the hospital phase of the study unethical because it withheld blood transfusion, the standard treatment for hemorrhagic shock, from some patients.[75]

Therapeutic clinical research has a responsibility to meet the standard-of-care—the normative standard that a qualified professional would use to manage the treatment. The ethical question raised with the PolyHeme trial was whether or not the in-hospital phase was a treatment that lay outside of the federal waiver, which allowed for exceptions only when an available treatment (in this case, the administration of whole blood) was unproven or not satisfactory. Nancy King and other bioethicists raised these concerns in an open letter about the trial: "For waived-consent trials, the patients/subjects must be in life-threatening conditions and proven, satisfactory treatments must be unavailable."[76] Whole blood, a satisfactory and standard treatment, was certainly available once these patients reached the hospital. Given this fact, on what basis did the PolyHeme trial pass IRB evaluation? How did this socially coherent group not raise ethical concerns about research on vulnerable populations?

One of the decided oddities of the trial was its "opt-out feature": people who knew about the experiment could call a local hospital that was participating and get a bracelet showing they had opted out of the trial, to wear in case they were the victim of an accident or injury and unable to speak for themselves. But as disturbing as the obstacles involved in "opting out" was the fact that the majority of the participating hospitals were urban medical centers that had a reliable population of patients who needed a transfusion. Because these patients would not be able to consent to a trial in the condition that would bring them to the hospital, the rule for a waiver of informed consent includes language that refers to a "community" consultation that replaces the gold standard of individual informed consent.[77] Given their central role as participants in the trial, it is not unreasonable to ask who the residents of these "communities" might be. How are their boundaries drawn? In the federal rules, "consultation" with a "community" displaces the direct consent of a single participant.[78] But who constitutes a community? Who is its legitimate spokesperson, and how does that spokesperson receive this authority? Dr. Eugene Dibble, then head of the John Andrew Hospital at the Tuskegee Institute, wrote to the president of the institute to urge its full participation in the syphilis study. Was his letter taken as "consent" for the men who were denied treatment for their disease? If so, by what ethical or legal authority did he speak for them?[79] The PolyHeme trials nearly mandated community participation. Only those who knew about the trial could opt out by calling a participating facility—an extraordinary feature for a clinical trial.

One area in which identities have come to matter in health science is the field of public health, as the U.S. public increasingly resides in urban areas, with growing minority populations. Minority city dwellers made up the community most likely to be included in the PolyHeme trial, which relied on big-city hospitals as a likely source of the patient population necessary for the study. Although Northfield did not explicitly state this reason (the company's website featured images of a traffic accident),[80] residents of cities are the most vulnerable to gunshot wounds, precisely the kind of injury for which PolyHeme might be administered. Given the contemporary ethnology of cities and gun violence,[81] it is not surprising that the populations for this trial come from inner cities, whose residents are predominantly black or brown. So for this trial, a subject's identity was not likely to be as random as the double-blind protocol—EMT specialists could not determine beforehand which of their transports would receive the blood substitute and which would not—implies.

When Surgeon General David Satcher wrote about community health in the *Yale Journal of Health Policy, Law, and Ethics*, he specifically linked the idea of community to racial and ethnic minorities and focused on health care disparities for these populations.[82] In public health parlance, "community" has generally come to mean populations who do not have access to private health care, who are generally nonwhite, and who live in urban environments. So when the federal rules use the language of "community" to suggest how an emergency medical waiver might be administered, the group of individuals for whom consultation displaces the practice of informed consent is unbalanced. It does not seem unreasonable to ask which bodies get to retain the gold standard of autonomous informed consent in medical practice, and which bodies are vulnerable to a waiver of this standard in order to advance emergency medical research. Picoult's Anna is biologically important to her family, a characteristic that displaces Anna's unique identity as well as overruling her autonomy. A similar intervention happens when a "community" stands in for an individual in medical research. There is no way to know the wishes of the individuals in such a situation. And there is no way to predict a common or shared consideration of an event such as a trial that waives informed consent. Is a community defined by boundaries of voting or school districts? What formulas assign someone the identity of member of a community? In amending a rule for informed consent with the idea of "community consultation," medical research proceeds on the fiction that a community is an identifiable and bounded construction that is similar enough to an individual research subject to be treated in the same regulatory manner.

Perhaps more than any other measure of identity, a community appears to be a public rather than private entity. This is the crux of the matter in the category of public health ethics, as well as in contemporary debates about a public option in the reformation of U.S. health care. The idea of a public includes certain kinds of bodies and excludes others. It is as much a class demarcation as it is gendered and racialized. In writing that "the existing formal codes and frameworks of bioethics [that] continue to give priority to *autonomy* [are] a poor fit for *public health* practitioners seeking ethics guidance for their *community-oriented* work" (emphasis added), the bioethicist Nancy Kass articulates precisely the ethical dilemmas involved in the field's distinctions between public and private, which award differential treatment to bodies depending on which domain they are assigned to.[83]

What ethical resolution would best protect a person's interest, given the acknowledged vulnerabilities of age (in the case of Anna), competence (in the case of traumatized or otherwise medically incompetent patients), or identity (inner-city residents), and that would balance the individual's rights with medical necessity? Readers of *My Sister's Keeper* confront competing interests that challenge the idea that the risks in this family's difficult circumstances can be resolved in a way that pays equal attention to each of the parties involved. And the complex family dynamics, ordinarily a private domestic challenge, are further complicated when they have to be mediated in public.

The idea of domestic privacy has long been a value in U.S. cultural history. It became a vigorously contested legal issue in 1890, when Warren and Brandeis argued the right to privacy as a legal tort.[84] One critical symbolic reference in their essay was its dependence on the implicit value of sanctity within the home. The idea of privacy as being reasonably located and embraced within the home was foundational to their claim.

Home was the romanticized location that the American poet Robert Frost wrote about in "The Death of the Hired Man": "Home is the place where, when you have to go there, / they have to take you in." Frost's sentiment underscores the idea of home as a sanctuary, a place where safety seems certain. A home's sanctuary and safety both extend from its privacy—from its protection from outside intrusions. Of the series of narratively critical settings in Picoult's novel—the hospital, the Fitzgerald home, the fire station where Brian Fitzgerald works, the lawyer's office, and the court—only one, the home, is presumptively private. Nevertheless, the other locations are where the family's most intimate decisions and crises are mediated, and each of those places is public. What happens to vulnerable populations when a home does not begin with that idea of a presumptive privacy, when a home is public housing?

A clinical trial that became a legal case, *Grimes v. Kennedy Krieger Institute, Inc.*, was a negligence claim brought by parents of minor children against the Kennedy Krieger Institute (KKI) in Baltimore, Maryland. KKI was a children's health facility affiliated with Johns Hopkins University. Between 1993 and 1995, KKI ran a nontherapeutic research study designed to determine the effectiveness of various levels of lead abatement in a public housing project. The U.S. Environmental Protection Agency was one of the funders of the study. Five categories of public housing received different levels of lead abatement. Families with children were eligible to be assigned to one of the three units of housing that were not completely cleared of lead, or to one of two control groups of housing—both of which had had full lead abatement procedures or had had no lead paint used in them. During the two years of the study, the

KKI took blood samples from the children to determine which levels of abatement were therapeutic. The study was designed to test samples at the initiation of the trial and at six-month intervals following the children's enrollment. It was also designed to refer children whose blood lead levels had increased by 5 μg/dL or children whose levels exceeded 20 μg/dL "for medical and environmental attention."[85] One of the claims of the Grimes lawsuit is that that protocol was breached on more than one occasion, with some children's unsafe lead levels left unreported for up to nine months. The court of appeals found for Grimes, stating that:

> Children . . . should not be enticed into living in, or remaining in, potentially lead-tainted housing and intentionally subjected to a research program, which contemplates the probability, or even the possibility, of lead poisoning or even the accumulation of lower levels of lead in blood, in order for the extent of contamination of the children's blood to be used by scientific researchers to assess the success of lead paint or lead abatement measures . . . [P]arents, whether improperly enticed by trinkets, food stamps, money or other items, have no more right to intentionally and unnecessarily place children in potentially hazardous non-therapeutic research surroundings than do researchers. In such cases, parental consent, no matter how informed, is insufficient.[86]

Ethicists were alarmed that the court ruling might mean a "challenge [to] the acceptable level of risk in pediatric research studies . . . that parents in the state of Maryland could not consent to their minor children's participation in research that posed even a minimal risk of harm if it offered no prospect of direct medical benefit to the subjects."[87] Although the court later clarified its initial decision, noting that a "minimal kind of risk is inherent in any endeavor" (an interpretation consistent with federal regulatory standards), the ethical outcry centered on the potential that this ruling had regarding the federal standard of minimal risk. The bioethicists focused on the loss of children from critical research paradigms. A cultural ethicist would have focused instead on the children who were the subjects in this study; their special vulnerability, given their qualification for public housing (an indication of their economic status and a likely indication of their ethnicity and race); and the errors acknowledged by the institute in reporting some of the dangerous lead levels.

Several factors made the children a "vulnerable" population. And either subsequently or coincidentally, their vulnerability rendered them available for public use as subjects in this trial. First, their homes were never invested with the sense of the private that motivated the privileged Boston lawyers who first claimed a legal right to privacy. The children's identities, as members of families whose incomes could not support private housing, literally rendered them available for this study. Their families were given incentives—"trinkets, food stamps, money," and so on, according to the court—to participate in the study. If signing a consent form for a study moves you into first place on the crowded rolls of those eligible for public housing, is this an incentive that compromises the validity of an ethically informed consent? Recall the consent given by parents of the Willowbrook children in order to have someone care for their youngsters' challenging mental disabilities. The idea of justice in ethics includes a principled neutrality—where decision makers as well as participants are free from any form of coercion that would compromise their participation.

When we consider the ways in which Anna's consent in Picoult's novel was won by her parents' desires, her sister's medical neediness, and the claims of kinship, we can see some parallels with a family enrolled in the Kennedy Krieger studies whose material needs might conflict with their desires.

A narrative like the fictional *My Sister's Keeper* brings out all of the thorny questions and thick contexts that exist in real medical cases. One important (if ultimately flawed) way that we read fiction is to look for the character or circumstances that most appeal to us—that are like those we have experienced, that we recognize, and sometimes, in a frequently heard phrase, "that we identify with." In fact, we bring some of these same reading biases to medical narratives. It is easy to see why such an approach, based on our own facility in identifying with a medical case, is flawed. But perhaps this novel's most important lesson for ethics is one reached through the device of the fictional perspective that allows, even encourages, an ethicist to confront the complexities of autonomy. Readers begin *My Sister's Keeper* cheering Anna's move toward emancipation—her effort to wrest the control of her body back into her own hands underscores her autonomy. Every move she makes in her pursuit of the intertwined goals of autonomy and emancipation seems right for a child who was raised to provide her sister with necessary biological products that would assure Kate's survival. However, when the reader discovers near the story's end that Kate has asked Anna to take up the legal battle for emancipation so that Kate can die in peace—she is tired of the exhaustive medical procedures—the reader has a responsibility to reassess the earlier judgment: Anna's attempt to separate her body from her sister's needs seems less brave and less autonomous. Instead of following her mother's directives, she is now following her sister's wishes. We don't learn what Anna would have wanted for herself. The complicated fact is that her self was successfully negotiated away from her early in the process of the medical procedures attached to her childhood. Reading *My Sister's Keeper* teaches us that autonomy is not in fact the neat ethical principle that bioethics would suggest it is. Instead, the complicated text of the novel's conclusion implies that autonomy may not be any more achievable within the institution of the family than it is within the institutional structures of medicine.

One of the lessons of narrative ethics is that we are likely to fall into the habits of reading a story when we read a case. Identity is precisely the variable that we should eschew, and yet it is often the one that is the most salient, the most recognizable. Identity matters complicate the terrain, whether we are reading fiction or encountering fact. Not only does identity render the private public, but in the narratives that lie within a clinical trial, the answer to "who's got the body?" is neither stable nor normatively coherent. It is this narratively dense terrain that medical ethics must acknowledge and negotiate in a clinical trial. Although an informed consent seems to be an adequate response to the question of autonomy, there are complications of identity—family, gender, maturity, race and ethnicity, and competency—that challenge the efficacy of a single form that reduces all participants to a common denominator.

FOUR

Immortality in Cultures

This chapter on death and dying considers the ways in which the principles of bioethics help us to negotiate events in medicine that affect the dying and their families. The idea of "unspeakable things unspoken" is the subtext of this chapter—knowing that the dead no longer have their voices and that what they would, or might, say is spoken by others whose own identities matter as they speak for the dead. "Immortality in Cultures" uses the lens of death and dying to examine the monumental and visible experiences during Hurricane Katrina, allowing that national memory to take its place in the critical context of biomedical ethics regarding death and dying. The primary literary reference in this chapter—a play, Margaret Edson's *Wit*—will recall the issue of clinical trials from the previous chapter, and the layers of narratives that construct the stories in *Private Bodies, Public Texts* will be relevant to the readings in this chapter that articulate the idea of a relationship between culture and immortality.

• • •

Children speak so powerfully in Jodi Picoult's novel, and the events of the novel so insistently surround their interests, that it is difficult not to consider them as the primary actors in the story. Who, finally, is *My Sister's Keeper*? The ordinary answer regarding a minor's keeper would be a parent. But the way in which the parents' diminished ethical responsibility fractures in the narrative places the autonomy of Sara and Kate in the foreground.

These sisters seem very different from another child—also with Old

Testament ties—and this time the story is of a father and son, Abraham and Isaac.[2] In that story from Genesis, Isaac's voice is only heard once: "Father?" "Yes, my son?" Abraham replied. "The fire and wood are here," Isaac said, "but where is the lamb for the burnt offering?"[3]

Readers already know two important points of context: there is an anticipated death, and that death will be considered an altruistic gift to God from Abraham, based on God's request. There is a similarity with Picoult's novel, where Anna is positioned by her parents—whose conduct is arguably God-like in terms of their presumptive authority to extend substance from her body as an altruistic gift to her sister. In these stories, sacrifice and death are not separate.

In medical ethics, narratives of the dying and the dead involve deeply intimate matters of relationship, sacrifice, loss, and even considerations of degrees of certainty around the embodied matters that the biblical story of Abraham and Isaac engages. The verses in Genesis suggest that Abraham did not hesitate to follow through with God's extraordinary demand to sacrifice his child, whom he arguably loved but not as much as he loved or feared the deity who demanded the gift. God rewarded Abraham's faith at the very last minute: just as the knife was poised above Isaac's flesh. He halted the sacrifice. But we are not privy to Isaac's voice at any point beyond that initial query. Is it important for a reader to consider Isaac's perspective regarding his father's faith and his own fate? Would it help our understanding of this story to know whether or not the child cried out with horror at the fate that was about to befall him? When the Lord enters into a conversation with Satan regarding God's servant, Job, the biblical language is intriguing: "Hast thou considered my servant Job?" The lexical use of "considered" is thick here. It implies a watchful regard, a notice, and a visibility that is not Job's prerogative to extend. In other words, Job's body is rendered into public service as an example of theistic fidelity, without his knowledge and without consideration of a principle like autonomy. The Lord and Satan both determine that Job's body will bear the public acts that will test his faith. And although Job does not die, the circumstances that extend from the Lord's "consideration" eventually mean that the center of the story becomes a question: Will Job speak? Will he curse God and die, or submit in silence?

When do the voices of the dying matter?

The relationship of the biblical story of Abraham and Isaac to issues in medical ethics is the intimacy of the relationship between father and child (arguably extended to God and God's "children") that, at the time one's life is ending, depends more on the relationship that will (arguably) be extant—that will survive any words spoken at the moment of the body's expiration. In reality, dying is a silent enterprise. This can happen because of the severity of the illness (because dying for many is preceded by insentience, like a coma), or because of the intervention of medical equipment, like a ventilator that permits mechanical respiration but prevents speech. Despite the hope that most have of dying with our loved ones surrounding us, at home, at peace, and without pain, many people die with only medical professionals who are strangers at their bedsides, in traumatic and painful exits from this life due to accidents, trauma, lethal lifestyles, or homicide. In fact, many people who die have as little opportunity as Isaac did to speak about their deaths.

In *How We Die*, a bioethicist and physician at the Yale School of Medicine, Sherwin Nuland, wrote: "Nowadays, very few of us actually witness the deaths of those we love. Not many people die at home . . . and those who do are usually the victims of drawn-out diseases or chronic degenerative conditions in which drugging and narcosis effectively hide the biological events that are occurring. Of the approximately 80 percent of Americans who die in a hospital, almost all are in a large part concealed, or at least the details of the final approach to mortality are concealed from those who have been closest to them in life."[4] Medical ethics has paid a significant amount of attention to the matters of death and dying, because of the finality of the moment—there is no opportunity left to revisit or to "consider" relationships, whether they are professional or personal—and also because the idea of medical futility is an area where negotiation between a patient, physician, and relatives is a normative protocol. The panic with which our culture often views this generally private conversation and decision making became publicly visible and highly incendiary in the summer of 2009, when the debate around a national health plan option included language regarding end-of-life determinations. When is it too late to treat a body? Who should determine the moment when medical intervention that is not palliative comes to a conclusion? What happens if we change our minds?

The ethics involved in death and dying also become public with regard to state death penalty policies. The ethical issues that matter in these cases begin with whether or not the death penalty is an ethical form of punishment, and if it is state policy, what role a physician should have in these state-mandated homicides. Is a physician's presence at an execution an "act"? Can a state medical board resolve these questions, or must the legislature settle them? In 2007 the North Carolina Medical Board adopted a policy that would discipline physicians who took an active role in executions. The question in North Carolina was whether the presence of a physician violated the medical ethics standard that ruled against "verbal or physical activity that . . . facilitates the execution."[5] The North Carolina Supreme Court determined that the medical board had exceeded its authority in ruling that physicians could not participate in executions. Associate Justice Edward Brady noted that for the board "to assert that the physician is to merely occupy space in a nonprofessional capacity is simply illogical and renders unintelligible the [state] requirement that 'the surgeon or physician of the penitentiary' be present."[6] Can a state mandate a physician's active role in executions—injecting the lethal drugs or monitoring respiration until it ends? The issues of cultural vulnerability that so readily attach to ethical issues addressed earlier in this book matter here as well. Those whom ethicists regard as vulnerable populations in considerations of clinical trials are also vulnerable in death penalty cases. Mentally impaired people, members of ethnic and racial minorities, and men are disproportionately executed, given their share of the population. And those convicted of homicide are more likely to be executed when the victims were white.

The novelist Ernest Gaines writes a compelling narrative about this kind of event in *A Lesson before Dying*. In the novel, a black man, Jefferson, is wrongly accused of murdering a white man during the course of a robbery. Jefferson's attorneys argue that he is so incompetent, the criminal complaint is unfair: "The public defender, trying to get him off, called him an animal . . . He said it would be like tying a hog down into that chair and executing him—an animal that didn't know what any of it was all about."[7]

The ethical abuses in the novel are legion, beginning with the conduct and decision of the legal system and extending to the cultural histories of the South (the novel is set in Louisiana); the narrative emerges in patterns that reinforce the importance of place. This is not a novel about whether or not Jefferson will be found innocent of the crime and freed. Instead, his death is a given. After rendering the matter of his innocence moot, Gaines focuses the reader's attention on the complexities of the culturally predetermined outcome and on the ethical complexities of Jefferson's inevitable execution. The narrative takes as its starting point the inevitability of the racialized outcomes attached to Jefferson's trial, his racial dehumanization, and the the grim ending. Grant Wiggins, a teacher, gives the condemned man a notebook and encourages him to use the few days he has left in life to write his own story. And it is because of the mental discipline required in the act of composition that Jefferson becomes less the farm animal that his own attorneys labeled him, and able to walk into the execution chamber as "the bravest man in that room."[8] His determined use of words to reclaim his humanity effectively erases the public defender's characterization of him. Jefferson's narrative acts—recorded in the notebook given to him by Wiggins—were transgressive as well as transformative. His writing displaces the official case document. Wiggins explains what he sees when Jefferson gives him the notebook to read:

> Jefferson had filled three quarters of the first page. The letters were large and awkward, the way someone would write who could barely see. He had written across the lines instead of above them. He had used the eraser so much that in some of the places the paper was worn through. Nothing was capitalized, and there were no punctuation marks. The letters were thin at the beginning, but they became broader as the lead was worn down. As closely as I could figure, he had written: *I dreampt it again last night. they was taking me some-*

where. I wasn't crying I wasn't begging. I was just going, going with them. Then I woke up. I couldn't go back to sleep. I didn't want to go back to sleep I didn't want to dream no more. There was a lot of erasing, then he wrote: *If I ain't notng but a hog, how come they just don't knock me in the head like a hog? Starb me like a hog?* More erasing, then: *Man walk on two foots; hogs on four hoofs.*

Later Jefferson writes directly to Wiggins:

Mr wigin you say rite somethin but i don't know what to rite an you say i must be thinking bout things i aint telin nobody an i order pout it on paper but i don't know what to put on paper cause i aint never rote nothin but homework i aint never rote a leter in all my life cause nana use to get other chiren to rite her leter an read her leter for her not me so i cant think of too much to say but maybe next time.[9]

Wiggins focuses so intently on the form and structure of Jefferson's writing ("across the lines," and "a lot of erasing") that he nearly misses the ontological question asked and answered in the first sample. Later, we see the ways in which Jefferson's writing traces the freedom of his own philosophical imagination. In one sense, it is represented in the opposition of the public and private prose ("you say rite somethin") and the difference between a more intimate, and arguably private speculation ("they say I'm nothin but a hog but. . . .").[10] Jefferson may not be formally lettered, but Gaines makes the evidence of his private spirit painfully and desperately apparent. *A Lesson before Dying* is not about Wiggins's assessment of Jefferson's writing, but of Jefferson's autonomy and his determined ownership of the narrative act.

Jefferson's successful displacement of the authoritative opening images of the courtroom with its protocol and recorded, official racism—the continuing execution of black men in Louisiana—is a narrative sleight of hand. The authorized documentary authority of the court becomes less important than Jefferson's own "unlettered" composition, which demonstrated the integrity and personal claim in his narrative so effectively that it belied the dispassionate history on display in the court. Jefferson's narrative manages to survive the constructed architectures of courtroom narratives, where the only defense imaginable would be one that stripped him of his humanity. He became what he wrote. At the novel's end his teacher, who had purposefully not attended the execution, heard its story: "'He was the strongest man in that crowded room, Grant Wiggins,' Paul said, staring at me and speaking louder than was necessary. 'He was, he was. I'm not saying this to make you feel good, I'm not saying this to ease our pain . . . I saw the transformation, Grant Wiggins,' Paul said . . . 'I'm a witness to that.'"[11]

Consider the lexical weight here, in the idea of a "witness." It is a legal term that is fully appropriate for this context. A witness is someone who can testify. A witness can be a part of an official record. At the end of a book that deals with the wrongful conviction and wrongful death of a black man, the man who "witnesses" the execution does not relate the story of the black man's dying, but instead gives witness to its complex lessons. This is the critical codicil to the story that could have been merely an official case record of the execution of a man who was wrongfully convicted. But Gaines insists that the story is instead a narrative of transformation—a salvific retelling of how a convicted criminal became a man in part because of the autonomy he claimed as his own narrator.

In this novel, the idea of narrative and story cannot simply mean the narrow legal execution of a text, or the medical record of a patient. Gaines suggests that transformation is the more capacious narrative act. In fact, it suggests that disciplinary authority might be an inappropriate frame. Jefferson's public execution was the only way his body gained a private personhood for him to claim. By the novel's end, he was fully human, having successfully escaped from the law's dehumanization. This was, of course, an extraordinary price to pay for a private and humane autonomy.

Robert Burt, a legal scholar and ethicist at Yale, explains that "the death penalty is the paradigmatic expression of officially sanctioned involuntary killing." He notes that "there is, moreover, no pretense of mercy."[12] Burt challenges the notion that a pretense of structural integrity conveys a protective neutrality: "The very structure of the administration of capital punishment depends for its moral legitimacy on a well-defined, self-conscious differentiation between 'guilt' and 'innocence.'

The rigidity . . . and the underlying, nagging implausibility of this differentiation is apparent in the . . . possibility that wrongfully convicted people might be executed."[13] After a provocative review of the history of death penalty legislation and its inconsistencies, including a trenchant commentary on abortion and the failure of the death penalty to meet the objective of rationality that otherwise guides judicial practice, Burt arrives at a conclusion that plunges us yet again into the complex interlocutions of the public and the private: "The need to differentiate between personal and official is a pervasive feature of social life, as is the similarly structured distinction between public and private realms."[14] Burt is inevitably Whitmanesque in his persuasive discussion of the relationship between death, law, and medicine, writing that "here is the paradox that we must somehow learn to live with in regulating death— that we must teach ourselves, through our rational intellectual capacities, that our rational intellect cannot adequately comprehend, much less adequately control death."[15]

Despite our desire and the ethical imperative to treat dying as one of the most sacred and intimate privacies of personhood, the event described in the introduction to this volume, the death of Terri Schiavo, became dramatically public. As Burt argues, our interests in regulation and rational intellectualism led to egregious violations of the humane principle that ought to have guided the public response—a respect for her privacy. Schiavo's dying was not only commented on by nonprofessionals, but it was intensely scrutinized by the media and was subject to political intervention. Florida's governor and state legislators and even the U.S. Congress tried to displace Schiavo's husband, Michael, from the role of decision maker on her behalf, as he sought to remove the ventilation tube that had been in place since the time of her automobile accident.[16]

Terri Schiavo's case is a contemporary text that ethicists frequently refer to in debates about a patient's right to die, the public's right to intervene, and the appropriate judicial role when these matters are contested. But it is interesting to consider Schiavo's case in the context of other infamous cases that have raised similar issues.

Constitutional privacy constrains the government's authority to intervene in personal choices. This includes the right for adults who are sufficiently capable of communication to refuse medical treatment, even if it would lead to their demise. The legal rights in these medical matters generally refer to the most basic of needs: nutrition (water and food) and ventilation. Both can be mechanically received (through ventilation tubes and gastric or nasal tubes). But persistent vegetative state (PVS) has sometimes made it difficult for a lay audience—notably a family—to determine that death has indeed occurred. Since a person in this state is not capable of communicating, medical professionals decide who can decide for the person whether to stop mechanical feeding and ventilating. If there is controversy regarding a hospital's determination of guardianship, the court steps in.

The first legal case involving PVS was that of Karen Ann Quinlan, a twenty-one-year-old New Jersey resident who consumed Darvon, Valium, and alcohol at a party and then collapsed at home. After three months of being supported by artificial ventilation and a breathing tube, her parents agreed with her physician's suggestion that the ventilator be removed.[17] When hospital administrators refused, the parents sued. Eventually the New Jersey Supreme Court ruled in their favor, noting that "it is the constitutional right of privacy that has given us most concern" and determining that "the State's interest . . . weakens, and the individual's right to privacy grows as the degree of bodily invasion increases."[18] The U.S. Supreme Court refused to hear the case. Karen Ann Quinlan's feeding tube was removed, and she died in 1985 in a nursing home as a result of pneumonia.

The Quinlan story riveted the attention of the U.S. public, press, and politicians throughout the period of the parents' dispute with the hospital. When Quinlan died, ten years after the final court ruling, the story was recirculated widely in the media.

The case was the subject of a television docudrama in 1976 and a cover story in *Newsweek* in 1975. In 1977, it was the impetus for sixty-seven bills introduced in state legislatures across the country regarding a patient's right to die.[19] In many ways it galvanized a public discussion of medical issues that would have remained private, had the hospital not disagreed with the parents' desires.[20] In addition, testimony at the trial indicated that Quinlan herself had expressed an opinion on the matter:

> Karen Quinlan is quoted as saying she never wanted to be kept alive by extraordinary means. The statements attributed to her by her mother, sister and a friend are indicated to have been made essentially in relation to instances where close friends or relatives were terminally ill. In one instance an aunt, in great pain, was terminally ill from cancer. In another instance the father of a girlfriend was dying under like circumstances. In a third circumstance a close family friend was dying of a brain tumor. Mrs. Quinlan testified that her daughter was very full of life, that she loved life and did not want to be kept alive in any way she would not enjoy life to the fullest.[21]

What were the constitutive elements that pushed this private issue into the public realm? The New Jersey Supreme Court's review of the case determined that Quinlan's right to privacy was implicated in decisions about whether to use medical equipment to prolong her life. As noted above, the court observed that "the State's interest *contra* weakens, and the individual's right to privacy grows as the degree of bodily invasion increases and the prognosis dims. Ultimately there comes a point at which the individual's right overcomes the state interest."[22] Is identity a consideration in this matter of privacy?

As we consider the answer to this question, work by Steven Miles and Allison August regarding gender, the courts, and the right to die is relevant. Their research determined that in "two of fourteen cases about profoundly ill women, courts ruled for the discontinuation of life-prolonging care. In eight similar cases involving men, no such orders were made."[23] The testimony of family and friends that the patient had stated no direct preference about care if he or she became medically incapacitated was more frequently accepted in cases involving men than in those involving women. In addition, the authors determined a linguistic choice that betrayed a gendered bias. Their research revealed that "women were referred to by their first names, and constructed as emotional, immature, un-reflective and vulnerable to medical neglect, while men were called by their last names, and constructed as ratio-nal, mature, decisive, and assaulted by medical technology. Only women were described as curled in a fetal position, while men were described as having contractures, the medical term."[24]

This evidence certainly suggests that gender matters in right-to-die cases. In fact, Miles and August's research ably predicted the courts' per-spective, discussed in this book's introduction, when it came to the case of Terri Schiavo, some eight years after their analysis was published.[25]

It is instructive to note which of these cases became media sensations, entering the public realm as obtrusively as the medical procedures in-vaded Quinlan's privacy, causing the court to refer to them as "bodily invasion."[26] Although the Quinlan court was referring to the mechani-cal devices that maintained her body after her brain function had sig-nificantly diminished, the language would apply to the treatment that Warren and Brandeis complained of in their *Harvard Law Review* essay. The authors wrote of the "inviolate personality" and "intrusions" that they expected personal privacy law would cover.[27] So in an important way, the convergence of tort law and constitutional rights centers on a person's body—and when the body belongs to a woman or a member of a racial or ethnic minority, the privacy these protections ordinarily grant is already at risk.

THE INTEXTUATION OF THE BODY

The Tuskegee syphilis study, whose protocols allowed men to die from a treatable disease, provoked significant changes in the national empha-sis and attention given to medical ethics. When this medical experiment became public in 1972 with a wire service story, and then a story in the *New York Times*, attention was focused on medical ethics as the field that ought to have prevented such events, given the Nuremberg Codes.[28] Fol-lowing the publicity about the Tuskegee study, the discipline of medi-cal ethics spent a substantial amount of time reassessing its attention to research trials and their processes. In 1997, the Institute of Medicine provided a valuable resource about end-of-life care that focused on im-proving that care. The publication included a critically important chapter called "Profile of Death and Dying in America," which reported data revealing the racial disparities in infant deaths and the ethnography of death in the United States. In other words, the report indicated where people die, as well as how—the actual physiological events that characterize a body's expiration. It also reviewed the legal issues that can emerge during these occasions, especially when there is a dispute between the patient, the patient's family, and medical institutions.[29] We have significant data from the sociology of death, the medical models of death, and the epidemiologies of dying in America. There is a wealth of aggregate data available from these sources and including trends and patterns that are geographically or racially informative. But aggregate data also formalize a priori presumptions.

Bioethics' attention to death and dying has focused on aggregate information. In one sense, narrative bioethics came about as a response to the data-driven information that delivered significant public-policy guidance but did not reveal the important stories behind the data. But categories of identity are relevant to these narrative ethics. The story of the Tuskegee syphilis study is actually a narrative about black men from an economic underclass who were victims of medical malfeasance. The response from bioethics to the eventually extraordinarily public tragedy of Tuskegee in many ways advanced the importance of a qualitative framing of medical matters. The structural guidelines of moral principles (autonomy, justice, nonmaleficence, and beneficence) gained force from a review of the tragedy of that medical experiment.

But what of the men who died at Tuskegee? What of the women who were subject to infection from the men's unrevealed syphilis, or their children born with the congenital form of the disease?

The bodies of those black men who died because of a failure to treat them have disappeared into relentlessly public national narratives of ethics in medicine, or into the cultural narratives that shared arguably idiosyncratic stories of medicine's neglectful or inattentive treatment to black Americans. Certainly the stories of the men and families who continued to live with this horror are as significant. The disease was passed on to wives and other sexual partners, and inherited by children as congenital syphilis. They became the invisible victims of this harm, and even today less attention has been devoted to these secondary infections than to the men who were the study's participants. But in this chapter's particular focus on the dead and dying, it is important to see how the narrative of the event was designed to excavate the bodies. The patients' personal privacy and intimate sexuality have been nullified each time some version of "what happened at Tuskegee" engages the public. And because race mattered in this medical event, the individual bodies of the patients were less important than the racial category that contained them. In this way, the very category of vulnerability that made them liable for ethical malfeasance also kept them relentlessly public. When identity matters, the individual is not as important as the collective. This is so especially when the collective represents a publicly noticeable body. Imagine being a black man today whose home is Tuskegee, Alabama—this story must resonate indeed. In fact, the death of a very prominent educator who founded the Tuskegee Institute, Booker T. Washington, was for many years presumed to have been related to syphilis, even though he was not a part of the official government study and although subsequent research has cast doubt on the syphilis diagnosis. There is dispute about the cause of his death related to the facts: his sexual conduct was gossiped about, his home was on the institute's grounds, and the doctor who examined him prior to death pronounced that his illness had decidedly "racial characteristics." That his consulting physician, Rufus Cole, was an expert on gonococcal infections certainly allowed the story of syphilis to taint this man's death.[30]

What might bioethics learn, then, from a single patient's story, or the individual narratives that have been recently heralded as the sine qua non of medical ethics?[31] It is certainly true that the field of bioethics might benefit from increased exposure to the categories of stories, theories of analysis, and the study of genre. But the relationship between a physician and a patient (the men of the Tuskegee study were both patients in the healthcare they ostensibly received from the clinic as an incentive to participate and subjects in the experiment) instinctively seems a more personal space, the space of the "patient versus body" binary from the anecdote I repeat in this book.[32] Nevertheless, what one discovers in stories are the thick public matters of culture and community—histories of families and social and political national stories that have their own meanings in the expansive sense of a speaker's meaning.[33]

Layers of meaning—even the contradictions of text that Walt Whitman acknowledged ("Do I contradict myself?")[34]—lie within and between the dramatic text of Margaret Edson's *Wit*, a play that depends on the interplay of bodies. The bodies are those of the patient, Vivian Bearing, an English professor who is dying of ovarian cancer; and two physicians who are medical researchers: Dr. Jason Posner, a former student of Professor Bearing's who studied poetry with her because "it looked good on my transcript to have taken her course,"[35] and his mentor, Dr. Harvey Kelekian. The two physicians are running what they anticipate will be a nontherapeutic clinical trial on an experimental cancer drug. Within the language of medical ethics, Bearing is effectively functioning as an altruistic donor, because the trial will not alleviate her disease—it has already progressed past the point of there being a cure. The donation of her body prior to her death for the physicians' assessment of chemotherapy dosages will assist in determining tolerable and therapeutic dosage levels for future patients and skews the ethics of patient care toward research objectives. Despite the insistently clinical narrative (recall the textual use of the word), Bearing, whose last name is surely a trope for the illness her body carries and the mantle it exacts, understands her physicians' microscopic interest in the nature of the cancer cells. Posner explains:

> You grow normal cells in a tissue culture in the lab, and they replicate just enough to make a nice, confluent monolayer. They divide twenty times, or fifty times, but eventually they conk out. You grow cancer cells, and they never stop. No contact inhibition whatsoever. They just pile up, just keep replicating forever. [*Pause.*] That's got a funny name. Know what it is? . . . Immortality in culture.[36]

Bearing is a Donne scholar, a critical theorist whose own version of the microscopic leads to her interest in the minutiae in Donne's texts—the intellectual conceits of puns, irony, and metaphor; the grammar; and the punctuation—which construct Donne's wit.

These constitutive parts of Donne's works, the parts that make up the body of his poetry and the imagery, are not lost in Edson's play, nor are they displaced from its subject. Language—even at its most basic level of words—is Bearing's defense. Her scholarly focus on Donne gives her a particularly intimate way of understanding her body's role in the unfolding drama of the end of her days. In fact, she is such a connoisseur of language that she looks up the medical terms that the doctors use. "It has always been my custom," she explains to the audience of the play (or to the readers of its text) "to treat words with respect."[37] The reader understands at this point that Bearing is being treated with less respect than the poetic words she has cherished during her professional career. In a contrapuntal interplay (the speeches occur simultaneously; in a staged performance, the lines would be delivered as if the other person were not speaking simultaneously) of her words addressed to the audience and the doctors' words addressed to gathered medical students, who view her as the specimen during grand rounds, Bearing explains the irony in a way that verifies her professional vision as well as argues for the potential contractive result of text, in Owen Barfield's terminology: "They read *me* like a book."[38] And the question of whether she is a patient or text produces the main tension of the play. The researchers push her to accept greater and greater doses of the drug—"Lower the dose? No way. Full dose. She's tough. She can take it."[39]—that is the focus of their nontherapeutic trial for the sake of medical knowledge, rather than for the remission of her disease.

When Kelekian, the senior physician on the research team, addresses Bearing directly, he appeals to what he presumes is their common appreciation of the gifts of mind, especially in his use of the pronoun "our" in noting that the increasingly painful and debilitating courses of chemotherapy will certainly be a tortuous course of treatment, but it is nonetheless necessary for her to endure them because, he notes, it "will make a significant contribution to our knowledge." Her reply—"Knowledge, yes"[40]—indicates that he has indeed touched on a common linguistic idiom. But the audience (or reader) knows that the two of them have no common value, no shared ethic. Kelekian's use of "our" is not about the cooperative effort between him and Bearing. In fact, her reply fails to use a determinative personal pronoun and simply declares the fact of "knowledge," as if the stark presence (and statement) of this word can encapsulate the unfolding drama of her death.

If a clinical trial does not represent the opportunity for a doctor and patient to exchange ethical values in a mutually agreed upon exchange of body for knowledge, or at the very least to agree about what will constitute the knowledge they seek, then what is it that binds the patient to this protocol other than the words of the contract—the informed consent that gives the protocol the right to proceed even up to the death of the patient? With dying patients like Bearing, what does altruism mean if the end of her body also holds an ethical conflict? She refers to the "'celebrity status' for the physicians 'upon the appearance of the journal article they will no doubt write about me.' But I flatter myself. The article will not be about *me*, it will be about my ovaries . . . my peritoneal cavity . . . What *we* have come to think of as me is, in fact, just the specimen jar, just the dust jacket, just the white piece of paper that bears the little black marks."[41]

Throughout the play, the reader comes to notice the similarities between Bearing's voice and the ironic poetic voice of Donne, who also contemplates the meaning of death and dying, and acknowledges his fear regarding the end of his life. In the passage above, perhaps the most pitiful irony lies in the line "what *we* have come to think of as me," indicating that her own sense of personhood, revealed as richly intellectual earlier in the play, has been reduced through the clinical protocol to text—the contracted vocabulary of medical print—not unlike the contracture of her own body into what lay persons identify as a fetal position. She lies curled into contraction—her own performance of diacritics—black marks without a critical reader attached. Consider the potential association here to Donne's "Hymn to God, My God in My Sicknesse":

> Whilst my Physicians by their love are growne
> Cosmographers, and I their Mapp, who lie
> Flat on this bed, that by them may be showne
> That this is my South-west discovery
> *Per fretrum febris*, by these straits to die.[42]

The lyrical idea of physicians as "cosmographers" and patients as the "map" recalls the metaphorical idea within "Cartographies of Desire," chapter 2 of this book. But notice who become the readers—the interpreters of the body's map. The identity of who is active and who is passive in Donne's sonnet mirrors not only the idea that the most intimate aspects of a body are like a map in terms of the body's legibility, but also the idea that a patient is subject to another's interpretive judgment, which—depending on what is at stake—may or may not be beneficent.

Medicine's most consistent effort—even within the science of genomics, but before that in biomedical research—is to discover ways to read the body. Between this act of reading and the patient's identity lies a legibility that is social, cultural, and political. Previous chapters of this book have explored the intersections of medicine and law as they attend to the body and as they make meanings out of some bodies that are attached to identity rather than simply being flesh. Abraham could not offer a lamb or any random body to the sacrifice. It was a particular flesh that God demanded of him, flesh that he loved: his own son. Identity matters, even in that biblical text.

The philosopher Michel de Certeau associates the different linguistic terrains that matter in terms of our regard for the body with their narratives. He explains that in writing, "normative discourse 'operates' only if it has already become a story, a text articulated on something real . . . i.e., a law made into a story and historicized . . . recounted by bodies . . . Every social orthodoxy . . . gives itself the form of a story and produce[s] the credibility attached to a discourse articulated by bodies."[43] De Certeau explains that flesh passes to "a word to become a fragment of language, a single name, that can be read and quoted." He names the process the intextuation of the body, which "corresponds to the incarnation of the law . . . For the law plays on it: 'Give me your body and I will give you meaning, I will make you a name and a word in my discourse.'"[44]

When bodies *make* "meaning" (when "Physicians . . . are growne Cosmographers"), they operate in linguistic systems that also regulate meaning—that assign certain words to certain bodies, or certain words to particular disciplines, all of which depend on their social circulations to share meanings across disciplinary boundaries. This is why it has be-

come so important to notice that bodies can operate as individual entities in medicine and law, but that corporate bodies become the focus in
medical ethics. The ways in which a body carries a story or text is significant inasmuch as it tells a reliable story about some body other than
its own. In these ways, identity matters.

Wit works not only because it rehearses the worst aspects of medical practice in terms of physicians' interest in and relationship to their
patients, but because the patient in this story is a woman, and her physicians are men. The gendered categories that Edson has assigned to the
drama's principal players matter in terms of their credibility. Bearing's
increasingly enfeebled state works as dramatic action not just because
the play is well written, but because she belongs to the category that the
legal analysis of Miles and August indicates results in different judicial
consequences in right-to-die cases, even to the extent of the court's language.

One reading of the story of Abraham and Isaac is that it is a precur-
sor to a story of God's own willingness to sacrifice his beloved son. In
that New Testament context, the story gains resonance: it is not simply
Isaac's helplessness that is the focus, but his eventual representation of
the sacrifice that Jesus executes—a body other than Isaac's is the rest
of the story. In that context, Isaac's symbolic presence matters; his identity as a son whose father is willing to sacrifice him is what is important
to the death narrative, rather than his being a child named Isaac. When
identity matters in law or medicine, the individual fades from the narrative, and a socially constructed body—one that matters in terms of its
representative potential—takes its place. This is why the stories of Karen
Ann Quinlan and Terri Schiavo, as individually compelling as each is,
can become a shared narrative regarding right-to-die cases and can also
represent the gendered dimensions of that story.[45] Even the cells that
so fascinate *Wit*'s Dr. Jason Posner were in fact (rather than the fiction
of the play) cells that replicated within the genetic substance of a black
woman, Henrietta Lacks, whose HeLa cell line is discussed in the introduction. Although Lacks's story is—like those of Quinlan and Schiavo—
important in its individual sense, the wrong perpetrated on her family
after her death is read into a narrative of black death and dying that has

made race matter. In fact, it is a narrative that makes black death a viable social construct despite the appeal of a value system that should argue against an associative nexus among race, gender, and conduct.

Despite our appropriate aversion to an association between identity and death, vital statistics point us precisely in that direction. Excess mortality—the phrase used to describe an incidence of death that exceeds statistical patterns of predictability based on known vulnerabilities (such as lifestyle, illnesses, and family background) is shaped within differences of culture or ethnicity. Foucault argues that this is a consequence of biopower, the authority of the state that determines and subsequently regulates differential value between its citizens and that makes "power . . . essentially what dictates . . . law."[46] This is the contemporary narrative implicitly rehearsed in genetic medicine's objective to discover factors that would make the patterns of disease vectors more predictable. But in the United States, race as socially constructed may be the result of genetic backgrounds, and it is further complicated by mixtures like that revealed in Chopin's "Désirée's Baby." How those categories are initially determined—and what are the social structures of those determinations—by scientists, who will later discern the meanings held within those categorizations, is as important as the outcome of the determinations.

When bioethicists consider matters of death and dying, they typically focus on the right to die, physician-assisted death, and palliation. As important as these issues are, the principle of justice draws our attention to matters of death and dying when social justice and inequity yield excess mortality in vulnerable populations. The bioethicists Madison Powers and Ruth Faden perceptively note that "inequalities in health that are a part of . . . systematic patterns of disadvantage are the inequalities that are most morally urgent to address. Justice here demands aggressive public health intervention to document and help remedy existing patterns of systematic disadvantage and their detrimental consequences."[47]

The courts' language regarding right-to-die cases illustrates the particularity with which women's bodies are viewed, at least in the law. A categorical (rather than individual) particularity reveals perceptual differences that are worthy of attention. At the very least, that is a failure of respect that has moral consequences at the moment of death and dying, which indicates how someone's private wish for dignity at the end of life is mediated by identity.

Powers and Faden advance a critical argument of moral urgency regarding identitarian inequities. They cite a study that "estimates that 886,202 deaths would have been averted if the mortality rates of African Americans and white Americans had been equalized in the decade from 1991–2000" and indicate that this kind of research indicates that "*public* acknowledgment that the failures of respect that underpin a web of negative determinants and consequences, including health inequalities, are unjust."[48]

DNR MEANS "DO NOT RESUSCITATE," NOT "DO NOT RESCUE"

In 2005, Hurricane Katrina slammed into the Gulf Coast of the United States, wreaking fatal havoc and leaving in its wake a horrific devastation—some produced by bureaucratic ineptness and inattention, and some by the failure of public health structures to manage a natural disaster of Katrina's proportions.

Narratives of the late-summer devastation are prolific and include books and academic articles as well as websites, films, and news reports. The voices in these stories include those of residents who found themselves stranded on rooftops, and who watched as everything from homes and automobiles to people and animals rushed past them mired in the fetid waters that continued to threaten their safety.

In downtown New Orleans, over six feet of water surrounded the Memorial Medical Center. Patients, medical professionals, family members, and survivors from the street attempted to find shelter in Memorial although the conditions there—suffocating heat with no power or water, and backed-up sewer lines—challenge the very idea of shelter. The historian Douglas Brinkley notes that "when people swam or paddled to the hospital seeking help, they were turned away. Memorial was in fact trying to evacuate its own patients."[49] Things were no better at Charity Hospital, "downtown New Orleans's huge depression-era monument to poor people's medicine."[50] At Charity, valiant battles raged to save the patients who were most in danger. Almost as an eerie irony, the rhythmic accompaniment to these efforts was the "whap whap" of army helicopters' rotors, which could be heard inside of Charity. Even as medical professionals worked in mounting desperation to protect the patients inside Charity, the public hospital, the army worked with similar determination to evacuate patients from the private hospital across the street, Tulane University Medical Center. "Everybody knew the score," reported one of Charity's physicians. "We had poor people. We were going to be last. Nobody had any illusions about that."[51]

When medical ethics takes note of vulnerable populations, it is important to remember that the members of these populations, if they are mature and physically competent, have as keen a sense of their own vulnerability as do the scholars who have assigned them to categories of reduced potential for equitable treatment in basic medical care. The emergency conditions that gripped New Orleans exacerbated the disadvantages of those categories, not only in terms of medical care but also in terms of the most basic humane treatment that ought to be common—indeed standard—practice in a democracy. In New Orleans during the days after Hurricane Katrina, the poor and black and elderly were particularly victimized by the tragic ineptitudes that followed in the storm's wake.

Once called Southern Baptist Hospital, the Memorial Medical Center was renamed in 1995 when Tenet Healthcare Corporation bought the property. Although the hospital was above sea level, because the whole city of New Orleans is low-lying, conditions there were dangerous after as well as during the hurricane. As long as the 260 patients remained inside, they were vulnerable to the extraordinary dynamics of the deteriorating conditions in the city. On the hospital's seventh floor were patients who were elderly or otherwise infirm residents of LifeCare, a long-term-care facility based in Plano, Texas, that leased the space from Tenet Healthcare. It was *not* a hospice floor: patients there were ill or injured and would eventually, after their conditions stabilized, be moved to rehabilitation or back to their homes. The conditions on the floor in the hours and days following the hurricane were horrendous in terms of the challenges to professional care and patient well-being. But few people would have anticipated that what happened to patients there would lead to murder charges being filed against a doctor and two nurses who were treating patients in LifeCare's leased facility.[52]

On Friday, September 2—six days after New Orleans mayor Ray Nagin issued his August 28 mandatory order to evacuate the city—the last of the staff was evacuated from Memorial. Nine days later, on September 11, forty-five bodies were removed from the filthy facility by the Disaster Mortuary Operations Team, mobilized after the hurricane by the National Disaster Medical System of the U.S. Department of Health and Human Services.[53] In the cases of four of the deceased removed from Memorial, Louisiana attorney general Charles Foti determined that the deaths were suspicious. His investigation followed news reports that there had been "mercy killings at Memorial."[54] These reports included the story of a CNN reporter's interview with Dr. Bryant King, who had been at Memorial "when conditions were at their worst":

> King said he is convinced the discussion of euthanasia was more than talk. He said another doctor came to him at 9 a.m. Thursday and recounted a conversation with a hospital administrator and a third doctor who suggested patients be put out of their misery.
>
> King said that the second physician—who opposed mercy killing—told him that "this other [third] doctor said she'd be willing to do it."
>
> About three hours later, King said, the second-floor triage area where he was working was cleared of everyone except patients, a second hospital administrator and two doctors, including the physician who had first raised the question of mercy killing.
>
> King said the administrator asked those who remained if they wanted to join in prayer—something he said had not occurred at the hospital since Katrina ripped through the city.
>
> One of the physicians then produced a handful of syringes, King said.
>
> "I don't know what's in the syringes . . . The only thing I heard the physician say was, 'I'm going to give you something to make you feel better,'" King said.

"I don't know what the physician was going to give them, but we hadn't been given medications like that, to make people feel better, or any sort of palliative care," he said. "We hadn't been doing that up to this point."

King said he decided he would have no part of what he believed was about to happen. He grabbed his bag to leave. He said one of the doctors hugged him.

King said he doesn't know what happened next. He boarded a boat and left the hospital.[55]

There were the kinds of similarities that bioethicists have categorized as vulnerabilities among the patients whose deaths were suspicious other than their assignment to the LifeCare floor. Many had do not resuscitate (DNR) orders—a designation not necessarily related to the predicted outcome of their hospitalization—and they were all black. The public deaths in New Orleans during and after the hurricane fit into a disturbing pattern of black death as a community narrative. Recall the odd interruption of the death of W. E. B. Du Bois's son in his classic *Souls of Black Folk*, where Du Bois writes that he and his wife walked behind the casket of their dead son in the streets of Atlanta and were assaulted with the shout of "nigger" from a passer-by.[56] The appearance of this private grief in the public stories of *Souls* seems an oddity, but one that can be explained by considering the incident "as much a public black story as were the powerfully provocative discursions on religion, music, freedom, and progress that framed other chapters in *Souls*," as I noted in an earlier work. The repetitive patterns of black death as a "color-coded death—the residue of riots, executions, suicides, and targeted medical neglect"[57] are part of the statistical fact of black death and dying in the United States. The circumstances of these patterns remove a significant potential of privacy from these deaths. They are presented publicly, either as statistics that fit into the categories of excess mortality among African Americans, or as the kind of story—like Terri Schiavo's—that turns the private event of dying into a public narrative.

Consider the story of the patients who died in New Orleans on the LifeCare floor in Memorial Medical. Media reports of euthanasia have incorporated however the patients died into the ethically fraught terrain of accusations of murder in the language of others—including those in the congregation of a local church to whom Eddie Jordan, the city's district attorney, spoke following the grand jury's decision that there was not enough evidence to pursue his petition for charges against the doctor. An ABC News online report carried the headline "Murder or Mercy at New Orleans Hospital?"[58]

The racial difference between the patients and the medical professionals frame the events of the story. Angela McManus had been at her mother's bedside night and day prior to the hurricane, and during its fury she slept in a bed next to her mother until the nurses indicated that her mother would be evacuated. It is not clear what amount of time passed before McManus discovered that her mother had not left the hospital as promised. So McManus "rushed back to the seventh floor," where she found her mother's condition had deteriorated:

"She was real lethargic . . . She would talk to me, then just doze back off. I was like, 'What's going on with her?' I was just sitting there talking to her and stroking her, and she was just sleeping and I'm like, 'Something is wrong.'"

McManus says nurses told her that her mother had been sedated. She grew concerned because she says her mother's pain had been manageable with Tylenol and an occasional painkiller . . .

Angela McManus became seriously frightened for her mother when she overheard nurses saying a decision was made not to evacuate LifeCare's DNR patients. "DNR means 'do not resuscitate.' It does not mean do not rescue, do not take care of," McManus said. She tried to rescind her mother's DNR order to no avail. On Wednesday evening, two full days after Katrina hit, Angela McManus says three New Orleans police officers approached her with guns drawn and told her she would have to leave. New Orleans police confirm that armed officers did evacuate non-essential staff from the hospital.

Confronted by police, McManus raced to her mother's bed. "I woke her up and I told her that I had to leave, and I told her that it was OK, to go on and be with Jesus, and she understood me because she cried,"

McManus recalled. "First she screamed, then she cried. And I said, 'Momma, do you understand?' And she said, 'Yes.' And she asked me, she asked me to sing to her one more time. And I did it, and everyone was crying, and then I left. I had to leave her there. The police escorted me seven floors down."

McManus says that when she left, only eight patients, including her mother, remained alive in LifeCare.[59]

That story of Angela McManus's mother's death, told to NPR in the context of its reporting on the alleged euthanasia or murder in the hospital during and after Katrina joins the narratives that become fully reasonable texts for medical ethics' focus on death and dying. Especially as the matter of euthanasia was debated after the hurricane, the idea of a mercy killing has especial resonance for medical ethics. Attention to the matter of euthanasia is certainly a predictable and not unreasonable focus for its academic and public-policy interests in death and dying. But the fact that these black patients also fit neatly into the category of those whom bioethics deems "vulnerable" indicates the story's reading into either the narrative of murder or that of mercy raises the event's potential to become a spectacle as well as draws the normative regard of ethics.

When we also consider the matter of the public narrative—whether it was of what happened specifically on the seventh floor of Memorial Medical, or what happened to a class of people including poor, black Americans in the days following the hurricane—the public blackness rehearsed during those days telescoped the histories of neglect or spectacular vulnerability attached to their identities. When the arguably ordinary (or at least predictable) questions of medical ethics regarding the principles of autonomy or justice are raised in these circumstances, it is difficult to separate them from the identities that regulate the frames of autonomy or the distributions of justice that might be relevant. What is the consequential difference between euthanasia and delivering morphine for palliative care when the patient will die from the effects of the drug on ventilation? Morphine slows breathing. Dr. Ewing Cook, a pulmonologist who had been appointed to the administrative team at

Memorial just weeks before the hurricane spoke to Sheri Fink, a physician at Harvard's Humanitarian Initiative who wrote an article for the *New York Times Magazine* a year after the storm. Cook said: "If you don't think that by giving a person a lot of morphine you're not prematurely sending them to their grave, then you're a very naïve doctor . . . We kill 'em." Fink wrote that "to Cook, the difference between something ethical and something illegal 'is so fine as to be imperceivable.'"[60]

Nonmaleficence? That very basic principle of ethical practice seems far removed from the dying in New Orleans. Justice? How to discuss that principle outside of the identities that mattered in New Orleans, not only during the days of the hurricane, but in whatever structures of practice would allow patients from a private hospital to reasonably anticipate an early rescue and render ordinary the assumption of those in charity wards that they would be last on the list? Although the hurricane provided a text to consider absolutely appropriate ethical issues like euthanasia and medical care, there was a text of black death and dying before the storm of death and dying at Charity—for instance, among New Orleans youth, or in the excess mortality of black babies. The attorney general's charges regarding the deaths at Memorial Medical were not supported by the grand jury. Eddie Jordan considered that outcome legally correct: "I think that the grand jury considered all the evidence, and carefully considered it." He added: "They concluded that no crime had been committed. And that is the decision of our grand jury, and I think justice has been served after due process."[61] The nurses, who had testified for the state, had been given immunity from charges.

The idea that there had been a governing regulatory process that implicitly guarantees the decision's credibility is not far removed from the physician's judgment in *Wit* that Vivian Bearing's chemotherapy was systematically correct. Events like her own pain and weariness, or even her memories, that might have intervened and attracted a compassionate attention to her as a person were subordinate to the protocol's regulations. Professor Bearing remarks: "Once I did the teaching, now I am taught." Who is the "I" in each clause of that sentence? Are they the same? As her body becomes text—a teachable thing—it also loses whatever claim it might have had to the kind of privacy, the intimacy of memory and desire, that an inviolable personhood would have been able to claim as judicious—to use a word that is intentionally evocative of the claims of Warren and Brandeis.

When Bearing finally dies, her former student, Dr. Posner, rushes to perform cardiopulmonary resuscitation (CPR), shouting orders to the nurse who screams back at him: "She's *no code!*" Posner finally realizes the orders do indeed say DNR (in another arguably gendered moment, he does not initially accept what the female nurse tells him, believing her only when she reminds him that he was there when the orders were signed by Dr. Kelekian). Posner whispers the play's final words: "Oh, God." It is a declaration that might be made toward the body that only moments before he had identified: "She's Research!" The capital *R* in the text of the play is an indication that for him, this is what her body is named. This is a proper and formal nomenclature that replaces "Vivian Bearing." But when he whispers "Oh, God," it follows his "howling" (according to the script) that *"I made a mistake!"*[62] So we don't know whether his divine appeal is because of his horror that he has made a medical error, with its potential professional consequences; or because of the trauma of the scene that has just ended, when he and the technicians violently assaulted Bearing's body with resuscitative measures that included pounding on her chest and delivering electric shock. Is he sorry for her or for himself?

We have learned enough through the play's unfolding of John Donne's poetry to consider Posner's appeal to the divine not unlike Donne's own agonies regarding death and the purposeful authority of the divinity. Is this the only proper regard of autonomy? Posner's appeal notably uses the very same language that Bearing utters in her own agony caused by the treatment. In fact, he witnessed his former professor's own petition: "Oh God. Oh God."[63] What does witness mean in this event? Is it enough akin to the medical idea of surrogacy that it should direct Posner's interest away from the clinical and toward the personal? The answer depends on what is lost (or gained) with Bearing's death. Lying before the audience in full public view are her evidentiary remains—ready to be plumbed once again, in autopsy. Is she a body, a patient, or "Research?" Is it a physical manifestation of Donne's metaphysical wit, his proposition that "gluttonous death" might have "instantly unjoynt [her] body, and soule"?[64]

In *Bodies That Matter*, the cultural theorist Judith Butler writes that "the matter of bodies will be indissociable from the regulatory norms that govern their materialization and the signification of those material effects."[65] Butler's is a compelling frame for understanding how the material regulations of the law, or medicine, construct the body as well as the meaning (the signification) that composes the consequential effect of that construction. Law and medicine are performances that regulate and constrain. Consider the public investment in the performative. As Bearing was reconstructed into a research subject (rather than a college professor) for Posner and Kelekian, she was physically and physiologically constrained by the requirements of the clinical trial. It regulated (or arguably became) her body's conduct. Nevertheless, at the play's end it is apparent that Bearing's insistently poetic voice is a syncopated accompaniment to the rhythm of the medical matters that control the narrative. Her voice, with its "wit" intact, inhabits the kind of private personhood that the clinical paradigm had displaced.

The bodies lost in New Orleans, when we remember them past those waning days of that summer tragedy, entered the public through images of horrific neglect during the days of flooding, and afterward as narratives that debated murder or mercy. The public story and its images provide substance for an ethical review of how the principles of medical ethics matter. Through the relentless public review of the circumstances and the maleficence that surfaced in the wake of the storm, private identities faded as black and poor victims were reconstructed into bodies whose personhood was performative, and whose narratives were relentlessly rehearsed in the chatter and print that followed the spectacular presence of the ends of their days.

Angela McManus's mother's name was Wilda Faye Sims-McManus. And although her daughter doesn't know the story of how or when she died, the immortal souls of Katrina have gathered themselves into a national narrative that weaves together the texts of this book—bioethics, medicine, and law. It is a story that will make its own meaning.

In 1933, the Harlem Renaissance author Arna Bontemps wrote a gentle and poignant story called "A Summer Tragedy," which chronicled the last hours in the lives of two elderly black sharecroppers, who realized their bodies were too frail for them to look after each other or to continue farming the land in a futile attempt to escape their indebtedness.[66] Bontemps reveals enough details to convince the reader of Jennie and Jeff Patton's significant illnesses and their age-related vulnerabilities (she is blind; he has had multiple strokes) as well as their economic insecurity. Once this background is clear, the story's placid pace belies the fact of their activity—a planned suicide—and the reader follows their careful final preparations with a breathlessness that anticipates the story's end.

Jeff and Jennie change into their best outfits, removing the ragged farm clothing that is their everyday wear and replacing it with a dress Jennie has put away for just this occasion and the "stiff-bosomed shirt" that Jeff will wear with a "swallowtailed coat . . . freshly brushed and pressed, but . . . as full of holes as the overalls in which he worked on weekdays."[67] Blind Jennie fumbles as she ties Jeff's bow tie, but after many years of marriage, she knows that he would never manage to get it quite right. The reader learns that they are alone in the world, having suffered the death of each of their five children in the two years before the story begins. Here, already the mark of black death intrudes as generational oxymoron when the reader notes that this elderly couple has had to bury their own children. The Pattons have no resources, they are facing final and terminal illnesses, and they have full and considered capacity to follow through with a plan long in the making. Bontemps writes that Jeff "could not bear to think of being helpless, like a baby, on Jennie's hands."[68] And Jennie could no longer see: "her useless eyes were wide and very white in their deep sockets."[69]

But even with the certainty of their decision, the narrative betrays its difficulty:

"You ain't really scairt, is you Jeff?"
    "Nah, baby, I ain't scairt."

"You know how we agreed—we gotta keep on goin'" . . .

"I don't know," he said with a shiver, "I reckon it's the only thing to do."[70]

Enough of the narrative is revealed for the reader to understand their plans, and to react with horror and pity at the loss—not only the impending loss of their lives, but the losses they have sustained through the forty-five years of their marriage.

Bontemps sets the locale carefully, in a manner similar to Ishiguro's careful descriptions of the English countryside in *Never Let Me Go*. Jeff and Jennie Patton emerge from their "tiny log house" into a day "warm and mellow with sunshine":

> Pine woods stretched away to the left like a black sea . . . Down the slope to the right were the cultivated acres on which the colored folks worked. They extended to the river, more than two miles away, and they were today green with the unmade cotton crop. A tiny thread of a road . . . ran through these green fields like a pencil mark.[71]

Bontemps marks the route to their dying as if it is a location on a map—as if it has, at least, cartographic familiarity. And the spirit the reader glimpses in them shimmers through the horror of their decision, sifts through some tears, and survives even some second-guessing as Jeff shifts his hat from one hand to the other and hears his wife's whisper "I'll soon be fixed to go."[72]

The language here recalls the archaic sense of "fixed"—as in stabilized, held in place—as well as the African American spiritual "Fix Me, Jesus." Indeed, the moments before the couple's passing are like the refrain from that spiritual, "fix me for my coming home—fix me, Jesus, fix me":

> Suddenly Jeff's hands became steady. He actually felt brave. He slowed down the motor of the car and carefully pulled off the road. Below, the water of the stream boomed, a soft thunder in the deep channel. Jeff ran the car onto the clay slope, pointed it directly toward the stream and put his foot heavily on the accelerator. The little car leaped furiously down the steep incline toward the water. The move-

ment was nearly as swift and direct as a fall. The two old black folks, sitting quietly side by side, showed no excitement. In another instant the car hit the water and dropped immediately out of sight.

A little later it lodged in the mud of a shallow place. One wheel of the crushed and upturned little Ford became visible above the rushing water.[73]

"A Summer Tragedy" exposes the contradictions and the pity of all the critical elements of narrative in bioethics: the duty of rescue and resuscitation, the inherent privilege of autonomy, and the complexity of public vulnerability. Death and dying are always stories of loss. These narratives, held in the fullness of time, expand and contract as if the certainty of our every breath might still the deafening silence of the missing. The waters of Katrina were not unlike the waters that took the lives of Jeff and Jenny Patton one tragic summer afternoon. Bontemps writes that "the years had fallen on them like waves."[74] What matters in fact, as well as in fiction, is act and intent. And sometimes the answer depends on the telling.

That same union of act and intent took place during the summer tragedy of Katrina. When waters and the times collide and then collapse, what's left is the visible tracery of tragedy. And, of course, the narrative cultures that expose its text, its subtexts, and what increasingly seems the inevitability of intersection.

CODA

In August 2009, Sheri Fink—an MD, a senior fellow at the Harvard Humanitarian Initiative, and a staff reporter at ProPublica—published one of the longest *New York Times Magazine* pieces in the paper's history.[75] It focused on the actions of Anna Pou, a doctor who remained with the patients on the LifeCare floor throughout the ordeal after the hurricane. Fink began her detailed and thorough review of the events at Memorial Medical with a particular focus—the conduct of Pou, whom the grand jury declined to indict after reviewing the district attorney's petition charging her with the homicide of four patients in particular, all of whom had received injections from her and all of whom had died, even though the illnesses that brought them to the hospital had not been life-threatening:

> The attorney general's office hired a forensic pathologist, Cyril Wecht . . . to review evidence in the deaths of four patients . . . Wecht concluded that all four deaths were homicides, caused by human intervention . . . Dr. James Young, the former chief coroner of Ontario Canada, who was then president of the American Academy of Forensic Sciences wrote in his report that "[a]ll these patients survived the adverse events of the previous days and for every patient on a floor to have died in one three-and-a-half hour period with drug toxicity is beyond coincidence."[76]

The grand jury took a host of factors into consideration, including medical reports—the case stories—as well as the narratives that were vigorously circulating among the general public.

But perhaps the most important narrative of the event is the one that has strained to remove itself from public consumption as it has framed and subsequently claimed a legal boundedness within the legislative back rooms where public policy is formulated. After the grand jury declined to follow the district attorney's request and issue an indictment, Pou dedicated herself to a very particular narrative—one constructed and bound by law. Fink explained:

> In the four years since Katrina . . . Pou has helped write and pass three laws in Louisiana that offer immunity to health care professionals from most civil lawsuits . . . for their work in future disasters, from hurricanes to terrorist attacks, to pandemic influenza . . . In her advocacy, she argues for changing the standards of medical care in emergencies. She has said that informed consent is impossible during disasters . . . The arguments she is making about disaster preparedness—that medical workers should be virtually immune from prosecution for good-faith work during devastating events . . .—are happening with little public discussion and insufficient scientific evidence.[77]

Informed consent, noted earlier as the gold standard of human subject research, which was already under fire by emergency medical waivers like those that allowed the PolyHeme trials to include an "opt out" clause, became Pou's focus. Another way to frame her efforts with regard to the standard of consent is to notice how they are specifically designed to remove these decisions from public circulation, to articulate them within the private enclaves of those professionals deemed to be the appropriate stakeholders, and to invoke—as did this book's introductory discussion of the distinction between the public and the private—the inviolate personhood that Warren and Brandeis imagined as inherent to a certain class of persons. An emergency would be enough to trigger the waiver that Pou advocates. But the logic that an emergency affects only the victims and not the medical professionals is belied in the narrative of post-Katrina New Orleans. All the people in the hospital—doctors, nurses, support staff, and patients alike—were affected by the stifling heat, the lack of air conditioning, fatigue, and mental exhaustion. An emergency is not selective in who needs care. What ethical credibility does the professional team have to remove consent from patients and turn it over to themselves, especially when their judgment cannot help but be compromised by mental and physical fatigue as that of everyone else involved in the emergency? The argument Pou has advanced is an ultimate example of paternalism, precisely the conduct that ethical codes of conduct were designed to remove.

In this particular case of contemporary legislative maneuvers, it would be medical professionals whose decision making about which lives to save would be absolutely and inextricably tied to the reality of social judgments about which lives are more valuable than others. Vulnerable bodies would gain no more protections from this kind of back-door protectionism than they already have in bioethics' beneficent notice of categories of caution.

Privacy circulates in complex and even contradictory ways in medical and legal texts. One thing is absolutely certain: vulnerable bodies, as soon as they are received into a category that urges an identitarian-based caution, are bodies whose flesh experiences what de Certeau explained as an "incarnation of knowledge . . . an intextuation."[78] Even the writing of a triage number (1, 2, or 3) that would determine their rescue and treatment status on patients' hospital garments—an event that actually occurred—or writing about the deceased victims captured in the ethical abyss of Memorial Medical, changed their flesh into vulnerable bodies— the kind of body that Vivian Bearing became, which was eventually read like a book; that could form the substantive claims of a district attorney's report of a crime; or that was at the center of my own discourse, when I described bodies' circumstances to the physicians at the lecture mentioned earlier in this book.

Despite, or perhaps because of, the intextuation, reconstruction matters greatly to narrative and to the culture constituting narrative's architectural scaffolding. The most consistent feature of textual bodies is the identity of which bodies are at stake in the claim to privacy, or violable by public relegation. During and after Katrina, the decisions made on the LifeCare floor of Memorial Medical or in the New Orleans convention center, or even in offices of the Federal Emergency Management Agency (FEMA), were made outside of public view. But the bodies that suffered the fleshly indignities in the New Orleans convention center or death due to toxic injections, or that were abandoned on rooftops or found floating on air mattresses through the foul waters of the flood were pitifully recognizable as belonging to the same bodily categories of vulnerability that bioethics claims is its consistent interest.

So what does a cultural bioethics do for our reading of these issues in medical ethics? First, it would do away with the claim that a patient's story, even if honored, could sufficiently frame or form a knowable product. A story is framed by the complexities of its cultural locations, even those that contradict themselves: by the forms of its telling, by those who speak, and by those who are spoken of. A cultural ethics would encourage serious and sustained attention to the kind of forecasting regarding national emergencies that might signal beforehand when bioethics' categories of vulnerability are themselves subjective categories that reveal as much about the field as they claim to reveal about a patient.

The cultural ethic embedded in the post-Katrina narratives is chilling and evident in two images of the disaster's aftermath, where different bodies negotiate the treacherous floodwaters. The photographs show people wading through the flooded streets. One image has an accompanying caption that says the white people in the photograph are wading through the water after "finding" food from a grocery store. The other image says the black man in the scene was "looting."[79] The only difference is race—and the language used to describe their parallel actions. The texts that accompanied these images were circulated worldwide and exhibited the pathological precision of intextuation subjected to another intextuation. A cultural bioethics knows, anticipates, and acknowledges the critical complexity in the rest of the text. In fact and in practice, bioethics is culture.

Notes

PREFACE

1. Among the many awards garnered by *Medical Apartheid* was the prestigious National Book Critics Circle Award for Nonfiction. However, the awards did not mute a fierce critique from a few voices in bioethics communities. See, for example, Ezekial Emmanuel, "Unequal Treatment," *New York Times Book Review*, February 18, 2007 (and Washington's response to Emmanuel's review, a letter to the editor published in the *New York Times Book Review*, March 17, 2007). Accompanying letters to the *Times* from Sheri Fink, a senior fellow of the Harvard Humanitarian Initiative, and Patricia Williams, a professor of law at Columbia University, take issue with Emmanuel's review. Washington's book provides an opportunity for sustained interrogation of the patterns of medical research. But (and it is perhaps *because* of these historical patterns that) the discipline of bioethics engages issues of race with some timidity and defensiveness, as reflected in some of the responses to Washington's text.

2. Foucault, *Psychiatric Power*, 44.

3. Ibid.

4. I refer here, of course, to Rita Charon's seminal work, *Narrative Medicine*. Charon's book encouraged medical professionals to receive "and understand what a patient goes through" (3). *Narrative Medicine* offers the idea of story to bioethics as a means of "bearing witness . . . [and] helping patients navigate the moral channels of illness" (203).

5. Butler, *Precarious Life*, xvii.

6. Ibid., 146.

1. Skloot, "Henrietta's Dance."

2. Ibid. Skloot continued her interest in this subject and published *The Immortal Life of Henrietta Lacks* in 2010.

3. Landecker, *Culturing Life*, 160.

4. Gold, *A Conspiracy of Cells*, 18.

5. Skloot, "Henrietta's Dance."

6. Van Smith, "Wonder Woman: The Life, Death, and Life after Death of Henrietta Lacks, Unwitting Heroine of Modern Medical Science," *Baltimore City Paper*, April 17, 2002 (http://www.citypaper.com).

7. Landecker, *Culturing Life*, 163.

8. Ibid., 164.

9. See, for example, the literary scholar Trudier Harris's essay "This Disease Called Strength," which explores the evolutionary stereotype of the overly strong, aggressive, indomitable black woman.

10. One of the most obvious problems for genomic science that might predict certain disease outcomes based on race is an African American patient whose race is socially constructed, and who would reflect a genomic history that indicates the complicated social histories of racial interactions in the United States.

11. This book's focus is on the United States, so "race" for blacks living in the United States will be captured with that imperfect nomenclature. It does not mean to dismiss the wide differences of geographies dispersed within the African diaspora—the Caribbean, Europe, and Canada, for example—that are held within the term *race*.

12. Rao, "Genes and Spleens," 377.

13. See Appiah, *The Ethics of Identity*, for a compelling analysis of identity, autonomy, and ethics.

14. Charon, *Narrative Medicine*, 3.

15. For a view of narrative bioethics, see ibid.; Charon and Montello, *Stories that Matter*; and H. Nelson, *Stories and their Limits*.

16. See Rothman, *Strangers at the Bedside*, for a history of the transformation in the American public's view of medicine, and of the influx of law and politics into the once insular domain of the physician.

17. Consider, for example, the tortured efforts on display during the Senate Judiciary Committee's hearings during the summer of 2009 regarding the nomination of Sonia Sotomayor to the Supreme Court. It was painfully difficult for some senators to separate her ethnicity from their gaze—as was most notably

and egregiously on display with Senator Tom Coburn (an Oklahoma Republican), who responded to her example of what a gun law might allow and disallow with a phrase popularized during the 1950s on the television show about a Cuban entertainer, Ricky Ricardo. "You have lots of splainin' to do," Coburn jokingly responded to Judge Sotomayor—who is Puerto Rican, not Cuban.

18. Rubenfeld, "The Right of Privacy," 744.

19. See Warren and Brandeis, "The Right to Privacy."

20. Rubenfeld, "The Right of Privacy," 753.

21. *Bowers v. Hardwick* was a 1986 U.S. Supreme Court decision that upheld the constitutionality of a Georgia sodomy law that criminalized consenting adults' private acts of anal and oral sex. The Supreme Court directly overruled *Bowers* in 2003, in *Lawrence v. Texas*, holding that the Georgia sodomy law was unconstitutional.

22. Warren and Brandeis, "The Right to Privacy," 195.

23. Lauren Berlant writes a cultural studies version of Rubenfeld's legal argument, noting that "privacy's fall from the utopia of normal intimacy finds the law articulating its subjects as public and American through their position within a hegemonic regime of heterosexuality, which involves coordination with many other normative social positions that are racially and economically coded toward privilege" ("The Subject of True Feeling," 126). Like Rubenfeld, Berlant argues that privacy becomes a cognizable legal issue in regard to sexuality.

24. I refer to this comment in *Codes of Conduct*, 3.

25. Appiah, *The Ethics of Identity*, 73.

26. In *The Ethics of Identity*, Appiah does indeed move directly to a consideration of autonomy following his discussion of "ethical individualism" in chapter 3, "The Demands of Identity." The difference I suggest here, in associating the ethics of identity with private autonomy, might be more a directional than a substantive difference from Appiah's argument.

27. The potential public exposure resident in these categories was particularly salient at the historical moment in the United States when political attention focused on Barack Obama as a black man and Hillary Clinton as a woman—both candidates for the Democratic Party's presidential nomination. Notice, however, that whiteness was erased for Clinton in the mainstream media's public discourse surrounding her candidacy—her race was not a category of spectacle; only her gender was the visible mark.

28. Of course there are times of ambiguity when race and women's gender are not evident. The argument about the spectacularity of these categories nevertheless holds, because these occasions are likely to spark even more public notice and queries about "what are you?" The biography of Anatole Broyard, former *New*

York Times Book Review editor, attracted a good deal more attention than it might have when it was disclosed that Broyard, who had lived his professional and personal life as a white man, was revealed to be black. See Gates, "The Passing of Anatole Broyard." Broyard's daughter wrote a memoir following her father's death that explores the history of her family and her own discovery and engagement with her mixed-race background (Broyard, *One Drop*).

29. William R. Levesque, "Schiavo's Wishes Recalled in Records," *St. Petersburg Times*, November 8, 2003 (http://www.sptimes.com).

30. Jenkins, *Private Lives, Proper Relations*, 20.

31. Although it is absolutely the case that the field of biomedical ethics has widely ranging theoretical interests, it is my assertion that even the claims in contemporary theories of bioethics have, at their root, an engagement with the traditional principles of the field—although the argument may be in favor of ultimately disengaging from these principles. So, for the purposes of this book, the principles of biomedical ethics—autonomy, nonmaleficence, beneficence, and justice—are the relevant place for its theories regarding privacy. See Beauchamp and Childress, *Principles of Biomedical Ethics*.

32. Barfield, *Speaker's Meaning*.

33. Holloway, *Passed On*.

I. BLOODCHILD

1. May, *Barren in the Promised Land*, 24 and 25.

2. Ibid., 37.

3. In reference to enslaved women, Deborah McGregor writes: "The political economy of slavery imposed a role on them defined by their ability to reproduce . . . In addition to the master's emphasis on reproduction, he would make frequent sexual demands of his own on slave women [that] figured into the rate of reproduction" (*From Midwives to Medicine*, 40).

4. Warren and Brandeis, "The Right to Privacy."

5. Ibid., 195.

6. See Alpheus Mason, *Brandeis*, especially chapters 4 and 5, "Boston: The Hub of the Universe and "The Brandeis Way of Life and Law," for a perspective into the class structures of Brandeis's intellectual and personal life.

7. Cooley, *The Law of Torts*, quoted in Warren and Brandeis, "The Right to Privacy," 193.

8. Warren and Brandeis, "The Right to Privacy," 195 and 215 for "inviolate personality," and 193 for "incorporeal" rights.

9. Kahn, "Privacy as a Legal Principle of Identity Maintenance," 372.

10. Ibid., 381.

11. Allen, *Uneasy Access*, 46.

12. Catherine MacKinnon notes that women's subordination happens because of the "private"—warning that "the distribution of power and resources within the private sphere will be precisely what the law of privacy exists to protect" (*Toward a Feminist Theory of the State*, 193). See also 184–94. Allen notes MacKinnon's perspective, juxtaposing it with a liberal feminist reconstruction of "decisional privacy" as an aspect of autonomy (*Uneasy Access*, 71).

13. Hill-Collins, *Black Feminist Thought*, 47.

14. *Roberson v. Rochester Folding Box Co.*

15. There is a substantial literature exploring issues of gender, reproduction, and privacy from a variety of perspectives. Some notable examples follow. Michie and Cahn's *Confinements* explores how a pregnant woman's body exposes her in particular ways in public culture, rendering her body a public battleground of reproductive choice despite the presumptive privacy of the domestic sphere. Inness's *Privacy, Intimacy and Isolation* is an invaluable exploration of the intersectionalities of privacy interests that begins with an acknowledgment that the word "privacy" provokes a chaotic responsiveness, precisely because of its reach and, ironically, our public interest in the private. Jenkins's *Private Lives, Proper Relations* considers African American literature's obsessive focus on a salvific self, a body and a reputation both preserved through propriety. Similarly, Shamir's *Inexpressible Privacy* focuses on fiction as a means of understanding the evolution of our contemporary understanding of privacy, conducting this interrogation through an interdisciplinary array of sources, from architectural drawings to literary texts. Helly and Reverby's *Gendered Domains* presents a series of essays that reexamine the oft-acknowledged gendered and separate spheres in which men's and women's history and labor contoured social understandings of the genders' roles. Allen's highly regarded *Uneasy Access* focuses on the gendered construction of the value of privacy. This interrogation is continued in Allen's *Why Privacy Isn't Everything*, where she focuses on the complex interplay of issues of race, family, health, and sexuality with regard to their correspondence with and disconnect from accountability.

16. Contemporary medicine understands vesicovaginal fistulas as a consequence of early birth—that is girls' giving birth before their bodies can normally accommodate labor—and of genital circumcision, a practice of some African communities that may have been unknown by plantation owners.

17. McGregor, *From Midwives to Medicine*, 61.

18. See also the discussion of Sims in chapter three. One relevant question here is why these enslaved women suffered this medical condition. Sims never

discusses how these women became pregnant, or the fate of the children these young girls bore.

19. See Lewis Wall's apologia for Sims in "The Medical Ethics of Dr. J. Marion Sims," 346–50.

20. Schwartz, *Birthing a Slave*, 5.

21. See Smedley, Stith, and Nelson, *Unequal Treatment*.

22. O. Butler, *Bloodchild and Other Stories*, 30. Butler thought that her readers' knowledge that she was African American contributed to their idea that the story was about slavery.

23. Ibid.

24. Ibid., 29.

25. Ibid., 6.

26. Ibid., 27–28.

27. See Johnson, *Griswold v. Connecticut*.

28. Henkin, "Privacy and Autonomy," 1410 and 1411.

29. Kate Chopin, "Désirée's Baby," 173–78.

30. Ibid., 174.

31. The skin darkening caused by melanin develops after birth.

32. "Visible admixture" was the nineteenth-century phrase that took on legal resonance with regard to denying persons of African ancestry equal rights with whites. For an example from Ohio of this kind of legislation, see Brown and Cayton, *The Pursuit of Public Power*, 182.

33. Chopin, "Désirée's Baby," 176.

34. Ibid, 177.

35. Ibid., 178.

36. The idea of a stain refers here to the genetic mark as well as the mark of social stigma.

37. See Garrow, *Liberty and Sexuality*, 195.

38. See Cheryl Harris, "Whiteness as Property," for a rigorous and original discussion of the association of property and race.

39. Chopin, "Désirée's Baby," 175.

40. "Rhinelander's Son Marries Daughter of a Colored Man," *New Rochelle Standard Star*, November 13, 1924.

41. See Lewis and Aridizzone, *Love on Trial*. Also note that Elizabeth Smith-Pryor's *Property Rites* (2009) explores the synergies between the contemporary culture, the legal and cultural ideas of property, and the spectacle of the Rhinelander heir in a public courtroom.

42. "Passing" for white was an option for people whose color was not discern-

ible, and that social phenomenon has been the subject of works of fiction (for instance by Nella Larsen) as well as of social science and legal scholarship.

43. See Onwuachi-Willig, "A Beautiful Lie," 2416, note 119.

44. Lewis and Aridizzone, *Love on Trial*, 59.

45. Onwuachi-Willig, "A Beautiful Lie," 2402.

46. Ibid., 2429.

47. Nothing in the court records indicate that the onlookers were directed to notice the color of her nipples. But there is no other explanation for this glimpse of her body—her arms and legs would have otherwise been a sufficient revelation.

48. Onwuachi-Willig, "A Beautiful Lie," 2429.

49. A composite image of Alice's disrobing is available online at the PBS website: http://www.pbs.org/ktca/americanphotography/features/digital/rhine lander_big.jpg.

50. Quoted in Washington, *Medical Apartheid*, 112.

51. See Jones, *Bad Blood*.

52. See Paul, *The Politics of Heredity*.

53. See DeLaet, *U.S. Immigration Policy in an Age of Rights*, and Haller, *Eugenics*.

54. Paul, *The Politics of Heredity*, 14.

55. Warren and Brandeis, "The Right to Privacy," 195.

56. Davis, "The Private Law of Race and Sex," 232.

57. Lewis and Aridizzone, *Love on Trial*, 13.

58. See Sartin, "J. Marion Sims."

59. Pernick, *A Calculus of Suffering*, 156.

60. Sims owned slaves, in his day referred to as "Africans"; the modern term "African American" implies citizenship, which these women did not have.

61. Sartin, "J. Marion Sims," emphasis added, 503.

62. Briggs, *Reproducing Empire*, 51.

63. Ibid., 108.

64. Linda Lewis Alexander, Judith H. LaRosa, Helaine Bader, Susan Garfield, and William James Alexander, *New Dimensions in Women's Health*, 92.

65. Gordon, *The Moral Property of Women*, 90.

66. De Arellano and Seipp, *Colonialism, Catholicism, and Contraception*, 116. Junod and Marks note that the Food and Drug Administration first approved the sale of Enovid at 10, 5, or 2.5 milligrams before settling on the two lower dosages ("Women's Trials," 143). These authors also give the history of contraceptive trials on the U.S. mainland and in England. In the United States, the trials were explained as research into gynecological disorders although "publications world-

wide had reported on Pincus's work and had speculated on the pill's clinical prospects" (ibid., 127).

67. De Arellano and Seipp, *Colonialism, Catholicism, and Contraception*, 116.

68. Vaughn, *The Pill on Trial*, 39.

69. Katherine McCormick quoted in Barbara Seaman, *The Greatest Experiment Ever Performed on Women*, 29 (emphasis added).

70. See Seaman, *The Greatest Experiment Ever Performed on Women*; Laura Briggs, *Reproducing Empire*; and Lara Marks, "A 'Cage' of Ovulating Females: The History of the Early Oral Contraceptive Pill Clinical Trials, 1950–1959," 221–48.

71. Roberts, *Killing the Black Body*, 94. See also Briggs, *Reproducing Empire*, especially chapter 5.

72. Roberts, *Killing the Black Body*, 95.

73. Moskowitz, Jennings, and Callahan, "Long Acting Contraceptives," S2.

74. See Roberts, "Punishing Drug Addicts Who Have Babies"; and J. Nelson, *Women of Color and the Reproductive Rights Movement*, especially chapter 2. Nelson's book explores the relationship between the feminist goal of a right to choose against the nationalist goal of having children "for the revolution."

75. Donald Kimelman, "Poverty and Norplant: Can Contraception Reduce the Underclass?" *Philadelphia Inquirer*, December 12, 1990.

76. The contraceptive effect of Norplant can last up to five years, but once it is removed, its impact fades.

77. "Sterilized: Why?" *Time*, July 23, 1973.

78. Kluchin, *Fit to Be Tied*, 100.

79. Ibid., 97. See also 97–101.

80. Karen Hawkins and Jeff Elliott, "Seeking Approval," *Albion Monitor*, May 5, 1996 (www.monitor.net).

81. Roberts, *Killing the Black Body*, 145.

82. Annas, "Fairy Tales Surrogate Mothers Tell," 48.

83. Roberts ("Punishing Drug Addicts," 1419) suggests privacy should be seen as the government's affirmative obligation to acknowledge a connection between the right of privacy and racial equality. The liberal (and feminist) construction of privacy as freedom from government restraints (a negative privacy) violates women's privacy rights.

84. MacKinnon has responded to privacy claims by noting that "the legal concept of privacy can and has shielded the place of battery, marital rape, and women's exploited labor," 101. See also Schneider, "The Violence of Privacy."

85. Davis, "The Private Law of Race and Sex," 224.

86. Even if his ancestry became public, he could have claimed assimilated whiteness. In *Tucker v. Blease*, the court found "void the marriage of a white per-

son with a negro or mulatto having one-eighth or more negro blood," but declared that "the child of a union of a white person and one having less than one-eighth negro blood is entitled to exercise all the legal rights of a white man, except those arising from a proper classification, when equal accommodations are afforded." Although this case was argued two decades after Chopin's 1893 short story, it was an indication that the law found a need to draw a line that would *prevent* too deep interrogations into the color line.

87. May, *Barren in the Promised Land*, 67.

88. *Daily Mail*, "My Ordeal, by Mother Who Had Black and White Twins," May 30, 2006 (http://www.dailymail.co.uk/health/article-388315/My-ordeal-mother-black-white-twins.html).

89. *Perry-Rogers v. Fasano*. See also Wiegman, "Intimate Publics, Race, Property and Personhood."

90. Bender, "Genes, Parents, and Assisted Reproductive Technologies," 4.

91. *Harnicher v. Utah Medical Center*.

92. Ibid., 69.

93. *Harnicher v. University of Utah Medical Center* (1998).

94. Baldassi, "Mater Est Quam Gestatio Demonstrat."

95. Vince, "White IVF Couple Have Black Twins."

96. Roberts, "Reconstructing the Patient," 120.

97. Ibid., 117.

98. Washington, *Medical Apartheid*, 64–65.

99. *Griswold v. Connecticut*, 485–86.

100. Warren and Brandeis, "The Right to Privacy," 220.

101. Allen, *Uneasy Access*, 72.

102. *Eisenstadt v. Baird*, 453.

103. Baldassi, "Mater Est Quam Gestatio Demonstrat," 6.

104. Mason and McCall Smith, *Law and Medical Ethics*, 57.

105. Ali and Kelley, "The Curious Lives of Surrogates," 114. Markens argues that media attention to surrogacy disputes (particularly the Baby M case) forced "political as well as public attention on surrogacy and initially helped define it as a social problem" (*Surrogate Motherhood and the Politics of Reproduction*, 22). Once surrogacy became a "social problem," governmental action ensued to regulate the process and the outcome.

106. De Certeau, *The Practice of Everyday Life*, 186.

1. Some researchers report a 99.5 percent similarity.

2. White House, Office of the Press Secretary, "President Clinton Announces the Completion of the First Survey of the Entire Human Genome: Hails Public and Private Efforts Leading to This Historic Achievement," June 25, 2000 (http://www.ornl.gov/sci/techresources/Human_Genome/project/clinton1.shtml).

3. White House, Office of the Press Secretary, "Remarks by the President, Prime Minister Tony Blair of England (Via Satellite), Dr. Francis Collins, Director of the National Human Genome Research Institute, and Dr. Craig Venter, President and Chief Scientific Officer, Celera Genomics Corporation, on the Completion of the First Survey of the Entire Human Genome Project," June 26, 2000 (http://www.ornl.gov/sci/techresources/Human_Genome/project/clinton2.shtml).

4. Ibid.

5. White House, "President Clinton Announces the Completion of the First Survey of the Entire Human Genome."

6. Ibid.

7. Legal cases have underscored the public-policy good of what would otherwise be a body's private property. The main precedent is *Moore v. University of California Board of Regents*, discussed in the introduction to this book.

8. Scholars and scientists have noted the public and private dimensions of this research, and some organizations, like Science Commons are working to create transparent documents of agreement for voluntary data sharing.

9. See, for example, the homo sapiens genome view at the National Center for Biotechnology Information's website: http://www.ncbi.nlm.nih.gov/mapview/map_search.cgi?taxid=9606.

10. The trilogy by J. R. R. Tolkien, *Lord of the Rings*, may be the most familiar example of fiction with this kind of illustration, which both mystifies and engages the reader, and serves as a guide to Tolkien's thickly populated stories with their many journeys.

11. I use "fanciful" here in its meaning creative, not decorative.

12. I use "illustration" here to mean something that renders another thing intelligible, or cognizable.

13. See Cavalli-Sforza and Feldman, "The Application of Molecular Genetic Approaches to the Study of Human Evolution."

14. White House, "President Clinton Announces the Completion of the First Survey of the Entire Human Genome."

15. A caution to the reader: the storyline of Ishiguro's novel is revealed almost immediately in this chapter.

16. Ishiguro, *Never Let Me Go*, 5–6.

17. Ibid., 159.

18. Ibid., 90.

19. Huxley, *Brave New World*, 11.

20. "Completing" is the euphemism for death in this novel.

21. Ishiguro, *Never Let Me Go*, 74.

22. Readers Read, "Interview with Kazuo Ishiguro," October 2005 (http://www.readersread.com/features/kazuoishiguro.htm).

23. I think here of "corporate" in its sense of corporeal, recalling the full physical body.

24. Reardon, *Race to the Finish*, 60–61.

25. See National Geographic Society, "The Genographic Project: Sample Results" (https://genographic.nationalgeographic.com/genographic/lan/en/sample_results.html).

Many twentieth-century American households kept and treasured old copies of *The National Geographic*—a magazine that connected them to parts of the world they might never visit, and that led them to value the projects of geography.

26. National Geographic, "About the Project," The Genographic Project (https://www3.nationalgeographic.com/genographic/about.html).

27. National Geographic, "How to Participate," The Genographic Project (https://genographic.nationalgeographic.com/genographic/participate.html).

28. The *New York Times* reporter Judith Miller was jailed for contempt of court for refusing to appear before a federal court with evidence regarding the identity of a CIA operative. Her appeal on the question of privilege, claimed as a First Amendment right, was heard in *In Re Grand Jury Subpoena, Judith Miller*. The court of appeals found the claim privilege overcome after determining the facts of the case. A *writ of certioriari* to the U.S. Supreme Court was denied.

29. Richard Cooper, Jay S. Kaufman, and Ryk Ward, "Race and Genomics," 1166. See also Reardon, *Race to the Finish*, 12.

30. Reardon, *Race to the Finish*, 60.

31. Including, for example, the history of the word "Caucasian"—originally a geographic term that now maps a conception of whiteness. I am grateful to Susan Reverby for pointing out this illustrative example.

32. Troy Duster, "Deep Roots and Tangled Branches," *Chronicle of Higher Education*, February 3, 2006, B13.

33. Ishiguro, *Never Let Me Go*, 81.

34. Ibid., 82.

35. Reardon, *Race to the Finish*, 5.

36. Variations in these human genes that are associated with tumor suppression have been linked to certain cancers—breast, ovarian, and prostate, in particular.

37. This is the problem with so-called orphan drugs—those pharmaceuticals associated with diseases that offer investors only little potential for great financial benefit.

38. Wailoo and Pemberton, *The Troubled Dream of Genetic Medicine*, 5.

39. The project is headed by George Church of Harvard University. It will publish the genotypes (and full names) of the volunteers, along with information about their phenotypes. The data will be posted on the Internet and will be free and accessible to all researchers interested in associations between genotype, phenotype, and environment.

40. George Church, interview by Diane Rehm, *Diane Rehm Show*, NPR, April 1, 2008. On a previous occasion, Church suggested that "as more and more of this kind of information becomes available, it will become more difficult to guarantee that it remains secure . . . Not only are 'hackers getting better at breaking through security,' said Church, but many researchers who gain permission to access de-identified data sets may unwittingly 'put it somewhere that Google can get to it.'" Understanding its vulnerability to hackers and public-use policies, Church suggested that "'we may need to start consenting to full disclosure' for all [private genomic sequencing] effort" (Bernadette Toner, "Harvard's Church Calls for Open Source, Non-anonymous Personal Genome Project," *Genome-Web Daily News*, November 14, 2005 [http://www.genomeweb.com/harvard-s-church-calls-open-source-non-anonymous-personal-genome-project]).

41. See, for example, Alondra Nelson's "BioScience Genetic Genealogy Testing and the Pursuit of African Ancestry" in *Social Studies of Science*, Vol. 38, No. 5. 759–83 (2008) and Charmaine Royal's "'Race' and Ethnicity in Science, Medicine, and Society." *Biosocieties*, 1 (3) 325–28 (2006).

42. See Lundy Braun et al. (2007), "Racial Categories in Medical Practice," 1423–28.

43. Quoted in "DNA Testing and Crime," *Religion & Ethics News Weekly*, May 28, 2004.

44. See Gordon-Reed, *Thomas Jefferson and Sally Hemings* and *The Hemingses of Monticello*.

45. Samuel Walker in the executive summary of a national survey of police DNA sweeps: Police Professionalism Initiative, "Police DNA 'Sweeps' Extremely Unproductive: A National Survey of Police DNA "Sweeps," Department of Crimi-

nal Justice, University of Nebraska, Omaha, September 2004. The report finds that DNA sweeps of possible criminal suspects to be "extremely unproductive" and recommended that "law enforcement agencies not conduct DNA sweeps based on general descriptions or profiles of criminal suspects." The report is available at http://www.unomaha.edu/criminaljustice/PDF/dnareport.pdf.

46. "CODIS is a computer software program that operates local, State, and national databases of DNA profiles from convicted offenders, unsolved crime scene evidence, and missing persons. Every State in the Nation has a statutory provision for the establishment of a DNA database that allows for the collection of DNA profiles from offenders convicted of particular crimes. CODIS software enables State, local, and national law enforcement crime laboratories to compare DNA profiles electronically, thereby linking serial crimes to each other and identifying suspects by matching DNA profiles from crime scenes with profiles from convicted offenders. The success of CODIS is demonstrated by the thousands of matches that have linked serial cases to each other and cases that have been solved by matching crime scene evidence to known convicted offenders" (DNA Initiative, "What Is Codis?" [http://www.dna.gov/uses/solving-crimes/cold_cases/howdatabasesaid/codis]).

47. Joh, "Reclaiming 'Abandoned' DNA," 860. Although one might have considered trash (garbage) one of the involuntary disposals that would ordinarily have a reasonable expectation of privacy, Joh's article cites *California v. Greenwood*, where the court held that there was no "reasonable expectation of privacy in trash bags left at the curb" because an item like a trash bag is "placed at the curb for the express purpose of conveying it to a third party . . . who might himself have sorted through the respondent's trash" (quoted in Joh, "Reclaiming 'Abandoned' DNA," 863–64). See also Holloway, Private Bodies/Public Texts and "Nothing's Secret."

48. Joh, "Reclaiming 'Abandoned' DNA," 862, note 26.

49. Ibid., 870.

50. The film is based on "Minority Report," a short story by Philip Dick.

51. Kittles and Royal, "The Genetics of African Americans," 226.

52. Ibid.

53. Ibid.

54. Ibid.

55. See Elliott, "Telling the Difference," 611 and 616.

56. *Doe v. Kamehameha Schools*, 1167. The three-judge panel of the Ninth Circuit originally overturned the district court's finding, but the review of the case set aside that panel's determination and upheld the legality of the schools' preferential admissions policy.

57. See ibid.

58. Kimberly Tallbear, "Narratives of Race and Indigeneity in the Genographic Project."

59. Indigenous Americans have so named the remains.

60. This theory of migration asserts that indigenous Americans are related to Asians who travelled across what is now the Bering Strait when it was land. Consider this point with regard to the Genographic Project's dependence on migratory patterns.

61. Consider the controversy engendered by "Bodies: The Exhibition," a show of bodies from China that toured the United States in 2005–7. The preserved, skinned, and partially dissected corpses were available for public viewing in cities across the country at a price set by exhibit coordinators.

62. Tallbear, "Narratives of Race and Indigeneity in the Genographic Project," 417.

63. Harry and Dukepoo, "Indians, Genes and Genetics," 8, quoted in Tallbear, "Narratives of Race and Indigeneity in the Genographic Project," 417.

64. Tallbear, "Narratives of Race and Indigeneity in the Genographic Project," 422–23.

65. Quoted in Brendan Koerner, "Blood Feud." Available at http://velielaw .com/showArticle.asp?articleid=45 and http://www.wired.com/wired/achive/ 13.09/seminoles.html.

66. See Bolnick et al., "The Science and Business of Genetic Ancestry Testing."

67. Gibson, "Long Way Home."

68. Ibid.

69. Other incidents of race-based ethical abuse include the gynecological experiments and surgery without anesthesia on slave women by Dr. J. Marion Sims (see chapter 1), the appropriation of dead slaves for medical research, radiation experiments on African Americans during the 1940s, and AIDS trials on black children in foster care without informed consent. For a history of these race-based medical practices, see Washington, *Medical Apartheid*.

70. Dayle DeLancey, "AIDSVAX & Artefacts: The Biomedical Industry, Clinical Trial Anomalies, and the Uses of African-American History in the Public Presentation of HIV/AIDS Vaccine Research," unpublished manuscript, University of Texas Medical Branch, 2008. See also, Brian Deer, VaxGen Company Reveals Some AidsVax Data—But Results Change from Show to Show," http://briandeer .com (http://briandeer.com/vaxgen/aidsvax-overheads.htm).

71. I am grateful to the bioethicist Dayle DeLancey for this example and reading of VaxGen's use of the Tuskegee narrative.

72. The drug's history is even more problematic. According to Jonathan Kahn,

"the developers of the drug test[ed] it in only one ethnic group [because] if the FDA had approved BiDil for the general population, the patent protection for the drug's manufacturer would have expired in 2007. Restricting the clinical trial to African-Americans maximized the chances that the FDA would approve the race-specific use of BiDil giving NitroMed an additional 13 years to sell the [drug] combination without competition" ("Race in a Bottle," 44).

73. It is not inappropriate to recall here the radiation experiments that led to U.S. blacks' receiving higher dosages of radiation during X-rays because of technicians' perception that their darker skin required more penetrating power.

74. Ishiguro, *Never Let Me Go*, 262–63.

75. White House, "Remarks by the President."

76. George Church, interview by Diane Rehm, *Diane Rehm Show*, NPR, April 1, 2008.

77. Ishiguro, *Never Let Me Go*, 266.

3. WHO'S GOT THE BODY?

1. For example, to study black males' vulnerability to prostate cancer, Rick Kittles and his colleagues used race and gender as significant variables in his research. See Kittles et al., "A Common Nonsense Mutation in *EphB2*."

2. For a thorough review of the Nuremberg trials and the evolution of the standard of informed consent in bioethics, see Weindling, *Nazi Medicine and the Nuremberg Trials*.

3. The U.S. National Institutes of Health, Office of Human Subjects Research, includes the Nuremberg Code on its website (http://ohsr.od.nih.gov/guidelines/nuremberg.html). See also Jones, *Bad Blood*; Washington, *Medical Apartheid*; and Reverby, *Tuskegee's Truths*.

4. See Holloway, *Passed On*, 82–88.

5. *Buck v. Bell*, 274 U.S. 200, at 270.

6. Ibid. See also the discussion in chapter 2 of the sterilization of women who were institutionalized or poor. The sterilization procedure was sometimes given the politicized name of "Mississippi appendectomy."

7. The eugenic focus on breeding—reproducing the most socially desired human beings—was practiced in part by classifying humans to isolate the mentally ill and infirm, people whose backgrounds were not Aryan (including Jews and blacks), and those who were not heterosexual. Early-twentieth-century birth control advocates paid specific attention to these social categories. Margaret Sanger, a prominent advocate for reproductive freedom, was also a founder of "The Negro Project," which advocated that racial purification was an appropri-

ate objective of birth control. See Franks, *Margaret Sanger's Eugenic Legacy*. To compare the association of disease with ethnicity, note the ways in which the psychological trauma of the Korean War was somatized regarding Puerto Rican veterans, who were described as having "hysteria," also known as the Puerto Rican syndrome. See Gherovici, *The Puerto Rican Syndrome*.

8. See Hornblum, *Acres of Skin*.

9. Retin-A, a drug used to treat acne, was a result of this experimentation. Dr. Kligman received the not insignificant revenue from its patent. In 2002, the Third Circuit ruled the statute of limitations had expired that would have allowed the class action lawsuit to proceed, and dismissed the case. The Holmesburg case is just one of a series of clinical trials conducted on incarcerated subjects.

10. One way that Southerners justified slavery was a cultural insistence that enslaved Africans were not fully human, and therefore had neither the emotional nor the intellectual capacity of whites. See, for example, William Wright's *Critical Reflections on Black History*, 36.

11. See Bosworth and Flavin, *Race, Gender and Punishment*. In their introduction to the volume, the editors write that "the widespread overrepresentation of minorities in penal systems that occurs around the world is nowhere more evident than in the United States." Citing 2005 statistics from the U.S. Department of Justice, they note that "since 1989, the number of black people incarcerated has surpassed that of whites, even though black men and women constitute only around 13 percent of the general population . . . [In] midyear 2004, 43 percent of the 1.9 million men in state or in federal prisons or in jail were counted as black" (Bosworth and Flavin, introduction, 1).

12. See, for example, H. Nelson, *Stories and Their Limits*.

13. Charon, *Narrative Medicine*, 3–4.

14. Jameson, *The Political Unconscious*, 185.

15. Indeed, it is unusual to see this field of narrative medicine emerge without substantive engagements that would liberate it from the sometimes laborious task of making something new, rather than participating in the helpful and substantial histories of literary theory. Its nominative gestures toward literary theory do not, as a rule, engage the history of those theories.

16. Whitman, *Leaves of Grass*, 83–86.

17. Ibid., 84.

18. Morrison, *Jazz*, 229.

19. Nussbaum, *Love's Knowledge*, 152.

20. This is a reference to a 2008 event that made headlines when Californian Nadya Suleman had octuplets by IVF, adding to the six children she had at home, also the result of IVF.

21. Tom Beauchamp and James Childress, *Principles of Bioethics*. See especially chapters 3–6, "Autonomy," "Nonmaleficence," "Beneficence," and "Justice," 57–282.

22. Anna Mastrioanni and Jeffrey Kahn, "Swinging on the Pendulum," 22.

23. From the 1950s to the 1970s, a research team at the Willowbrook State School for the mentally retarded intentionally infected children with hepatitis in order to study the natural course of a disease that they presumed would eventually affect children who were hospitalized in the unsanitary conditions that prevailed at Willowbrook. There was a waiting list for admission, and parents' consent to their child's participation meant a speedier admission to the school. The ethical question would regard the exploitation of consent for parents who were frantic for some remedial care for their children. See Katz, *Experimentation with Human Beings*, 1007–10; and Goodman and McElligott, *Useful Bodies*.

24. See *Hyman v. Jewish Chronic Disease Hospital*. Chester Southam, a physician at Memorial Sloan-Kettering Cancer Center, injected twenty-two elderly residents at the Jewish Chronic Disease Hospital with cancer cells to determine whether people without cancer, but who are debilitated, would reject cancer cells more quickly than cancer patients. The patients were not told the injections contained cancer. See also Katz, *Experimentation with Human Beings*, 9–65.

25. Mastroianni and Kahn, "Risk and Responsibility," 1074.

26. Anna Mastroianni and Jeffrey Kahn, "Swinging on the Pendulum: Shifting Views of Justice in Human Subjects Research," *Hastings Center Report* 31, no. 3 (2001): 22.

27. When "experiment" is used lexically, the focus is generally on the abuse of the study, rather than a neutral explanation of its procedures.

28. See Reverby, *Examining Tuskegee*, for a current and thorough history of the culture and the consequences of the study.

29. Mastroianni and Kahn could simply have assumed the reader would be so familiar with the Tuskegee study that they did not need to give information about its population and ethical breach, as they did in the other two "exemplary" cases of ethical breaches.

30. For patients with syphilis not enrolled in the study, penicillin became the drug of choice for treatment in 1947. The study withheld this treatment from its subjects until its negligence was exposed in 1972.

31. In one study of why black women received lower doses of a treatment than white women, the researchers concluded that "we know little about the structural causes for these disparities," but they did not include an interrogation of medical bias. See M. Sorbero, A. Dick, and J. Griggs, "Racial Variations in Adjuvant Chemotherapy Regimens for Breast Cancer," presented at the

AcademyHealth meeting in San Diego, California, 2004 (http://gateway.nlm.nih .gov/MeetingAbstracts/ma?f=103624332.html).

32. The Comstock Act, passed in 1873, prohibited the distribution of contraception, pamphlets, or other literature that explained contraception or research into birth control methods.

33. Quoted in Wald, *Contagious*, 114.

34. Ibid., 115.

35. In a discussion of "one-strike" policies from the U.S. Department of Housing and Urban Development, Mele notes that "residents . . . forgo unfettered rights of association and privacy of social relations . . . In turn, the cost of being poor, black, and a resident of public housing is a decreasing level of privacy over one's everyday life" (*Civil Penalties, Social Consequences*, 136).

36. This history is perhaps most forcefully illustrated in the application of the death penalty in the United States for the crime of rape. The only criminal conduct that did not involve the killing of another human being that could earn the death penalty was rape. And this penalty was specifically associated with black men convicted of raping white women. Rise describes a 1951 case as the "earliest instance" of using statistical evidence, history, and sociology to prove systematic discrimination against African Americans in criminal cases (*The Martinsville Seven*, 99). These men were executed for the crime of rape despite the fact that no white man had ever been sentenced to death for rape in Virginia, in records that dated back to 1908 (ibid., 119 and 120). See also Ifill, *On the Courthouse Lawn*.

37. There is a long and distinguished history of the emergence of public health in the United States. See Farmer, *Pathologies of Power*; Finkel, *Truth, Lies, and Public Health*; and Wald, *Contagious*.

38. Picoult, *My Sister's Keeper*, 3.

39. Ibid., 3, 19.

40. The first letters of the girls' names are phonologically similar to Cain and Abel. Notice, though, that Picoult has switched the initial phonemes of who kills whom—or has she?

41. Picoult, 31.

42. Ibid., 169.

43. It is also important to consider here in what ways the uses of altruistic donation—the gift—is gendered.

44. Picoult, *My Sister's Keeper*, 54.

45. Ibid., 144.

46. Ibid., 102–3.

47. Washington points out the error of such categorizations, noting that "His-

panic is an ethnic category, encompassing people of white, black, and mixed race" (*Medical Apartheid*, 272).

48. Ibid.

49. Pine et al., "Platelet Serotonin," 538 and 539.

50. Washington, *Medical Apartheid*, 272. Discussion of a "warrior gene" proves that the history of words conveys particular social paradigms ("'Warrior Gene' Predicts Aggressive Behavior After Provocation," *ScienceDaily*, January 23, 2009 [http://www.sciencedaily.com/releases/2009/01/090121093343.htm]).

51. Glantz, "Nontherapeutic Research with Children," 238.

52. Washington, *Medical Apartheid*, 275.

53. Personal conversation with Dr. Leslie Clapp, senior medical director, Medical Affairs Novella Clinical Research Organization, November 13, 2009.

54. 21CFR50 Subpart D.

55. The 2004 survey included 4,005 Americans and was funded by the Pew Charitable Trusts. Of those surveyed, 57 percent disapproved of using PGD for sex selection, and 80 percent "were concerned that if not regulated, reproductive genetics technologies such as PGD could 'get out of control'" ("Genetic Testing of Embryos to Pick 'Savior Sibling' OK with Most Americans," *Medical News Today*, May 4, 2004 [http://www.medicalnewstoday.com/articles/7899.php]).

56. Altman's *Who Goes First?* is a fascinating exploration of physicians and scientists who use their own bodies for research. The book does not focus on the ethics involved, but it does directly address the question of whether clinical trials must involve large populations.

57. Mastroianni and Kahn, "Swinging on the Pendulum."

58. Sims, *The Story of My Life*, 269. The discussion of Sims in chapter 1 of this book focuses on the reproductive dimensions of his experimentations and the lack of an expectation of privacy for slave women.

59. Ibid., 326.

60. Ibid., 327.

61. Wall, "The Medical Ethics of Dr. J. Marion Sims," 349.

62. Rosser, *Women's Health*, 91–92.

63. Chasnoff, Landress, and Barrett, "The Prevalence of Illicit-drug or Alcohol Use during Pregnancy."

64. Roberts, *Killing the Black Body*, 175.

65. Rosser, *Women's Health*, 86.

66. See the World Medical Assembly website and the evolving statements of the Helsinki Declaration at http://www.wma.net/en/30publications/10policies/b3/index.html.

67. Marlene Cimons, "CDC Says It Erred in Measles Study," *Los Angeles Times*, June 17, 1996. Although some have suggested that Satcher's own identity matters (he is African American), I fail to see its relevance here. He acted in his capacity as head of the CDC. It is particularly interesting that one of the characteristic responses to claims of race or gender bias is that the perpetrators are themselves black or women, and therefore could not be acting in a racist or sexist way. But in fact, biases are perpetrated by all kinds of people with power. There have been slave traders who were native Africans, Africans in America who owned slaves, and black policemen who used excessive force (or stood by while it was used) on suspected criminals. Bias is about power, and whoever wields the power can act out of a society's normative social script.

68. Ibid.

69. Washington's *Medical Apartheid* devotes a significant number of pages to these trials, and commentary is also available online.

70. Faden and Beauchamp, *A History and Theory of Informed Consent*, 277 (emphasis added); see also 176–277.

71. Ibid., 277.

72. Between 1988 and 2001, over 400 children in foster care, believed to be HIV-positive, were enrolled in a New York City study of HIV/AIDS drug regimens. After a public outcry regarding the enrollment of the children, the majority of whom were black or brown, in a "drug experiment" that linked the ethics of the case to Tuskegee, an independent agency, the Vera Institute of Justice, was commissioned in 2005 by New York City's Administration for Children's Services to examine the enrollment and monitoring of the New York City children enrolled in the study. The Vera Institute's final report, released to the media on January 28, 2009, noted that "while the child welfare agency had developed a policy in the late 1980s, the regulations were not always followed. For example, some children participated in trials that were not approved by the child welfare commissioner, files were poorly managed and often incomplete, and informed consent documents were often missing or filled out incorrectly. In some cases, child welfare files described deviations from the processes required by federal regulations and Children's Services policy, and Vera reviewers found that three children had been enrolled in a Phase 1 trial that had not been approved by the child welfare commissioner." Vera Institute of Justice, "Vera Institute Releases Final Report on NYC Foster Children in Clinical Trials for HIV/AIDS," January 28, 2009 (http://www .vera.org/news/vera-institute-releases-final-report-nyc-foster-children-clinical-trials-hivaids).

73. Faden and Beauchamp, *A History and Theory of Informed Consent*, 277.

74. See FDA Code of Federal Regulations 21 CFR 50.24. (http://www .accessdata.fda.gov/scripts/cdrh/cfdocs/cfcfr/CFRSearch.cfm?fr=50.24).

75. See Kipnis, King, and Nelson, "An Open Letter to IRBs Considering Northfield Laboratories' PolyHeme Trial." See also Holloway, "Accidental Communities."

76. Kipnis, King, and Nelson, "An Open Letter to IRBs Considering Northfield Laboratories' PolyHeme Trial," 20.

77. Code of Federal Regulations Title 21, Vol. 1 (http://www.accessdata.fda .gov/scripts/cdrh/cfdocs/cfcfr/CFRSearch.cfm?fr=50.24).

78. The federal regulation states that research conducted under §50.24 (7.i) requires "consultation . . . with representatives of the communities in which the clinical investigation will be conducted and from which the subjects will be drawn" (http://www.accessdata.fda.gov/scripts/cdrh/cfdocs/cfcfr/CFRSearch .cfm?fr=50.24).

79. Thanks to Susan Reverby for providing that example regarding the letter from Dr. Dibble.

80. Northfield Laboratories, Inc., "Potential Uses for PolyHeme" (http://www .northfieldlabs.com/uses.html).

81. The U.S. Department of Justice reports that twice as many blacks as whites die by gun violence in the United States (http://bjs.ojp.usdoj.gov/content/homi cide/race.cfm).

82. Satcher, "Our Commitment to Eliminate Racial and Ethnic Health Disparities."

83. Kass, "Public Health Ethics," 235.

84. Warren and Brandeis, "The Right to Privacy."

85. See Buchanan and Miller, "Justice and Fairness in the Kennedy Krieger Institute Lead Paint Study," 783. See also Mastroianni and Kahn, "Risk and Responsibility."

86. *Grimes v. Kennedy Krieger Institute, Inc.*, 814.

87. Mastroianni and Kahn, "Risk and Responsibility," 1073. An alternative view, expressed in a personal correspondence (September 19, 2010) with Nancy Kass is that "for researchers to try to make a horrid situation better does not . . . make them deserving of criticism. . . . Clearly more fundamental solutions are needed, but public policy decisions repeatedly suggest that disadvantaged populations are not going to be helped in these more fundamental ways and often public health comes in to see if shorter-term solutions that might, actually, be implemented, are effective."

1. Morrison, "Unspeakable Things Unspoken."

2. The allusion for the Picoult novel is the Old Testament story of Cain and Abel.

3. Genesis 2:23.

4. Nuland, *How We Die*, 8.

5. The board's statement is that "any physician who engages in any verbal or physical activity . . . that facilitates the execution may be subject to disciplinary action by this Board. See "North Carolina Medical Board's Position on Capital Punishment" at http://www.ncmedsoc.org/non_members/regulatory/NCMB_capital_punishment.pdf.

6. *NC Dep't of Corr v. NC Med Board* (51PA08), May 1, 2009, at 21.

7. Gaines, *A Lesson Before Dying*, 31.

8. Ibid., 260.

9. Ibid., 229.

10. Ibid., 222.

11. Ibid., 260.

12. Burt, *Death Is That Man*, 123.

13. Ibid., 124.

14. Ibid., 139.

15. Ibid., 185.

16. See Blendon, Benson, and Herrmann, "The American Public and the Terri Schiavo Case"; and Racine, Amaram, Seidler, Karczewska and Illes, "Media Coverage of the Persistent Vegetative State and End-of-life Decision-making."

17. Quinlan's mother wrote that the feeding tube remained in place until the daughter's death (Quinlan, *My Joy, My Sorrow*, 38).

18. *In re Quinlan*, 355 at 41.

19. See McDougall and Gorman, *Euthanasia*, 7. Only eight of these bills became law.

20. Burt presents a compelling and thoughtful discussion of this case, including the difference between the public's perception of it—that physicians wanted to prolong Quinlan's life at any cost—and the truth of the matter: her physician, Fred Plum, explained at the trial, to an inattentive court, that "she did not need a respirator to survive" (quoted in *Death Is That Man*, 15).

21. *In re Quinlan*, 348 at 801.

22. Ibid., 355 at 41.

23. Miles and August, "Courts, Gender and the Right to Die," 85. The authors reviewed twenty-two cases from appellate courts in fourteen states to arrive at

their finding that a gendered bias was discernible in the courts' ruling with regard to these cases.

24. Ibid., 88.

25. The case of Terri Schiavo began in 1998, when her husband petitioned the court in Pinellas County, Florida, to remove the feeding tube that had been in position since 1993.

26. *In re Quinlan*, 355 at 41.

27. Warren and Brandeis, "The Right to Privacy," 195.

28. Jean Heller, "Syphilis Victims in U.S. Study Went Untreated for 40 Years," *New York Times*, July 26, 1972. Susan Reverby's important recent study (*Examining Tuskegee*) makes the critical point that Heller's exposé came at the right time and place to attract attention to racial disparities in the United States. These disparities were not irrelevant to the attention the story received.

29. Field and Cassel, *Approaching Death*.

30. I note in an earlier work that the "injudicious airing of the characteristics of his illness encouraged an unfortunate private speculation" (Holloway, *Passed On*, 116). Susan Reverby notes the correlation between Washington's professional location and the narrative of his illness writing that Washington's successor at Tuskegee was "acutely aware of what was presumed to be the extent of the disease and its ties to assumptions about black immorality" (Reverby, *Examining Tuskegee*, 39–40). Although syphilis is no longer suspected as the cause of his death, in 1915, when he died, the rumor was already planted when Washington's own physician contributed to the speculation about syphilis in his oblique reference to "racial" reasons for Washington's final illness. By the time of the syphilis experiments at Tuskegee, the events of Washington's illness and the syphilis experiment settled into complementary narrative ground.

31. See Charon, *Narrative Medicine*.

32. In chapter 1 of *Useful Bodies*, "Making Bodies Useful: Historicizing Medical Experiments in the Twentieth Century," Goodman, McElligott and Marks acknowledge the shifts that happen between patients and subjects, especially with regard to the bodies of black patients who constitute vulnerable subject populations. They note that informed consent was the mechanism ethics proposed to address this potential overlap, but that there are, nevertheless, examples that indicate the boundaries are less easy to maintain when "patient" care is a part of clinical trial protocol (*Useful Bodies*, 4). In Gilbert Whittemore and Marilyn Boleyn-Fitzgerald's contribution to that volume, these authors perceptively ask, "in what way [are] the subjects of experiments useful bodies? . . . They were patients whose bodies were used" ("Injecting Comatose Patients with Uranium: America's Overlapping Wars Against Communism and Cancer in the 1950s," 166).

33. See Barfield, *Speaker's Meaning*.

34. Whitman, *Leaves of Grass*, line 1321.

35. Edson, *Wit*, 30.

36. Ibid., 56.

37. Ibid., 41.

38. Ibid., 37 (emphasis added). See Barfield, *Speaker's Meaning*.

39. Edson, *Wit*, 45.

40. Ibid., 11.

41. Ibid., 53.

42. Donne, "Hymn to God, My God in My Sicknesse," 211. *Per fretrum febris* means "in a feverish state."

43. De Certeau, *The Practice of Everyday Life*, 149.

44. Ibid.

45. Perspectives on end-of-life care have shifted, especially after the public rehearsal of Schiavo's death. See Hampson and Emanuel, "The Prognosis for Changes in End-of-Life Care after the Schiavo Case"; and Emanuel, "A Review of the Ethical and Legal Aspects of Terminating Medical Care."

46. Foucault, *The History of Sexuality*, 83. Foucault explains that "the subjugation and control of populations mark[ed] the beginning of an era of 'biopower.'" 140.

47. Powers and Faden, *Social Justice*, 87.

48. Ibid., 89 (emphasis added). The study cited is Steven H. Woolf et al. "The Health Impact of Resolving Racial Disparities" (2008): 26.

49. Brinkley, *The Great Deluge*, 481.

50. Horne, *Breach of Faith*, 130.

51. Ibid., 138.

52. See *State of Louisiana v. Anna M. Pou, Lori L. Budo, and Cheri A. Landry* (http://news.findlaw.com/hdocs/docs/katrina/lapoui706wrnt.html).

53. Brinkley, *The Great Deluge*, 635.

54. Jamie Wilson, "Allegations of Mercy Killing in Hurricane Aftermath," Guardian.co.uk, October 15, 2005.

55. Kathleen Johnston, "Staff at New Orleans Hospital Debated Euthanizing Patients," CNN.com, October 13, 2005.

56. Holloway, *Passed On*, 5.

57. Ibid., 3.

58. "Murder or Mercy at New Orleans Hospital?," July 19, 2006, ABCnews .com.

59. Carrie Kahn, "New Orleans Hospital Staff Discussed Mercy Killings," *All Things Considered*, February 16, 2006.

60. Fink, "Strained by Katrina," 8.

61. Russell McCulley, "Murder Charges Dropped against Katrina Doctor," Reuters, July 24, 2007.

62. Edson, *Wit*, 84.

63. Ibid., 70.

64. Donne, quoted in ibid., 52.

65. J. Butler, *Bodies That Matter*, 2.

66. Bontemps, "A Summer Tragedy." In Abraham Chapman, ed. *Black Voices*, 87–96.

67. Ibid., 88.

68. Ibid., 94.

69. Ibid., 92.

70. Ibid.

71. Ibid., 89.

72. Ibid.

73. Ibid., 96.

74. Ibid., 95.

75. Fink, "Strained by Katrina."

76. Ibid., 45.

77. Ibid., 30.

78. De Certeau, *The Practice of Everyday Life*, 143 and 149.

79. The first photograph was taken by Dave Martin for the Associated Press on August 30, 2005. The caption reads: "A young man walks through chest deep flood water after looting a grocery store in New Orleans on Aug. 30, 2005." The second photograph was taken by Chris Graythen for AFP/Getty Images, also on August 30. The caption says: "Two residents wade through chest-deep water after finding bread and soda from a local grocery store after Hurricane Katrina came through the area in New Orleans, Louisiana." These images are available online at Jed Morey's Blog in a post from January 21, 2010, titled "White Men Can't Jump . . . or Loot" (http://jedmorey.files.wordpress.com).

Bibliography

Books and Articles

Alexander, Linda Lewis, Judith H. LaRosa, Helaine Bader, Susan Garfield, and William James Alexander. *New Dimensions in Women's Health.* 5th ed. Sudbury, Mass.: Jones and Bartlett, 2010.

Ali, Lorraine, and Raina Kelley. "The Curious Lives of Surrogates." *Newsweek,* April 7, 2008, 45–52.

Allen, Anita. *Uneasy Access: Privacy for Women in a Free Society.* Lanham, Md.: Rowman and Littlefield, 1988.

———. *Why Privacy Isn't Everything: Feminist Reflections on Personal Accountability.* Lanham, Md.: Rowman and Littlefield, 2003.

Altman, Lawrence. *Who Goes First? The Story of Self-Experimentation in Medicine.* Berkeley: University of California Press, 1998.

Annas, George J. "Fairy Tales Surrogate Mothers Tell." In *Surrogate Motherhood: Politics and Privacy,* edited by Larry Gostin, 43–58. Indianapolis: Indiana University Press, 1988.

Appiah, Kwame Anthony. *The Ethics of Identity.* Princeton: Princeton University Press, 2005.

Baldassi, Cindy L. "Mater Est Quam Gestatio Demonstrat: A Cautionary Tale." Working paper, June 27, 2007 (http://ssrn.com/abstract=927147).

Barfield, Owen. *Speaker's Meaning.* Middletown, Conn.: Wesleyan University Press, 1967.

Beauchamp, Tom L., and James F. Childress. *Principles of Biomedical Ethics.* 5th ed. New York: Oxford University Press, 2001.

Bender, Leslie. "Genes, Parents, and Assisted Reproductive Technologies: ARTs,

Mistakes, Sex, Race, & Law." *Columbia Journal of Gender and Law* 12, no. 510 (2003): 1–76.

Berlant, Lauren. "The Subject of True Feeling: Pain, Privacy, and Politics." In *Left Legalism/Left Critique*, edited by Wendy Brown and Janet Halley, 105–33. Durham: Duke University Press, 2002.

Blendon, Robert J., John M. Benson, and Melissa J. Herrmann. "The American Public and the Terri Schiavo Case." *Archives of Internal Medicine* 165, no. 22 (2005): 2580–84.

Bolnick, Deborah A., Duana Fullwiley, Troy Duster, Richard S. Cooper, Joan H. Fujimura, Jonathan Kahn, Jay S. Kaufman, Jonathan Marks, Ann Morning, Alondra Nelson et al. "The Science and Business of Genetic Ancestry Testing." *Science*, October 19, 2007, 399–400.

Bontemps, Arna. "A Summer Tragedy." In *Black Voices: An Anthology of African American Literature*, edited by Abraham Chapman, 87–96. New York: Signet, 2001.

Bosworth, Mary, and Jeanne Flavin, "Introduction: Race, Control and Punishment: From Colonialism to the Global War on Crime." In *Race, Gender and Punishment: From Colonialism to the War on Terror*, edited by Mary Bosworth and Jeanne Flavin, 1–12. New Brunswick, N.J.: Rutgers University Press, 2007.

Braun, Lundy, Anne Fausto-Sterling, Duana Fullwiley, Evelyn M. Hammonds, Alondra Nelson, William Quivers, Susan Reverby, and Alexandra Shields. "Racial Categories in Medical Practice: How Useful Are They?" *PLoS Medicine* 4, no. 9 (2007): 1423–28.

Briggs, Laura. *Reproducing Empire: Race, Sex, Science and U.S. Imperialism in Puerto Rico*. Berkeley: University of California Press, 2002.

Brinkley, Douglas. *The Great Deluge: Hurricane Katrina, New Orleans, and the Mississippi Gulf Coast*. New York: Harper Perennial, 2007.

Brown, Jeffrey Paul, and Andrew Lee Cayton. *The Pursuit of Public Power: Political Culture in Ohio 1787–1861*. Kent, Ohio: Kent State University Press, 1994.

Broyard, Bliss. *One Drop: My Father's Hidden Life; A Story of Race and Family Secrets*. New York: Little, Brown, 2007.

Buchanan, David and Franklin Miller. "Justice and Fairness in the Kennedy Krieger Institute Lead Paint Study: The Ethics of Public Health Research on Less Expensive, Less Effective Interventions." *American Journal of Public Health* 96, no.5 (May 2006): 781–88.

Burt, Robert. *Death Is That Man Taking Names: Intersections of American Medicine, Law and Culture*. Berkeley: University of California Press, 2002.

Butler, Judith. *Bodies That Matter: On the Discursive Limits of Sex*. New York: Routledge, 1993.

————. *Precarious Life: The Powers of Mourning and Violence*. London: Verso Press, 2004.

Butler, Octavia E. *Bloodchild and Other Stories*. New York: Seven Stories, 1995.

Cavalli-Sforza, Luigi, and M. W. Feldman. "The Application of Molecular Genetic Approaches to the Study of Human Evolution." *Nature Genetics Supplement* 33 (2003): 266–75.

Charon, Rita. *Narrative Medicine: Honoring the Stories of Illness*. Oxford: Oxford University Press, 2006.

Charon, Rita, and Martha Montello, eds. *Stories That Matter: The Role of Stories in Medical Ethics*. New York: Routledge, 2002.

Chasnoff, Ira. J., Harvey J. Landress, and Mark E. Barrett. "The Prevalence of Illicit-drug or Alcohol Use during Pregnancy and Discrepancies in Mandatory Reporting in Pinellas County, Florida." *New England Journal of Medicine* 322, no. 17 (1990): 1202–6.

Chopin, Kate. *Bayou Folk*. Boston: Houghton, Miflin and Company, 1894.

————. "Desirée's Baby." In *"The Awakening" and Selected Stories of Kate Chopin*, edited by Barbara Solomon. New York: Signet Classic, 1976.

Cooley, Thomas. *A Treatise on the Law of Tort or the Wrongs Which Arise Independent of Contract*. 2nd ed. Chicago: Callaghan and Co., 1888.

Cooper, Richard S., Jay Kaufman, and Ryk Ward. "Race and Genomics." *New England Journal of Medicine* 348, no. 12 (March 20, 2003): 1166–70.

Davis, Adrienne. "The Private Law of Race and Sex: An Antebellum Perspective." *Stanford Law Review* 51, no. 2 (January 1999): 221–88.

de Arellano, Annette Ramirez, and Conrad Seipp. *Colonialism, Catholicism, and Contraception: A History of Birth Control in Puerto Rico*. Chapel Hill: University of North Carolina Press, 1983.

de Certeau, Michel. *The Practice of Everyday Life*. Translated by Steven Rendall. Berkeley: University of California Press, 1984.

DeLaet, Debra L. *U.S. Immigration Policy in an Age of Rights*. Westport, Conn.: Praeger, 2000.

Donne, John. *Poems of John Donne*. Vol 1. Edited by E. K. Chambers. London: Lawrence and Bullen, 1896.

DuBois, W. E. B. "Of the Passing of the First-Born." In *The Souls of Black Folk*, 169–75. New York: Penguin, 1989.

Elliott, Michael. "Telling the Difference: Nineteenth-Century Legal Narratives of Racial Taxonomy." *Law and Social Inquiry* 24, no. 23 (1999): 611–36.

Emanuel, Ezekiel J. "A Review of the Ethical and Legal Aspects of Terminating Medical Care." *American Journal of Medicine* 84, no. 2 (February 1988): 291–301.

Faden, Ruth R., Tom L. Beauchamp, and Nancy M. P. King. *A History and Theory of Informed Consent*. New York: Oxford University Press, 1986.

Farmer, Paul. *Pathologies of Power: Health, Human Rights, and the New War on the Poor*. Berkeley: University of California Press, 2004.

Field, Marilyn J., and Christine K. Cassel, eds. *Approaching Death: Improving Care at the End of Life*. Committee on Care at the End of Life, Institute of Medicine. Washington: National Academy Press, 1997.

Fink, Sheri. "Strained by Katrina, a Hospital Faced Deadly Choices." *New York Times Magazine*, August 25, 2009 (http://www.nytimes.com/2009/08/30/magazine/30doctors.html).

Finkel, Madelon Lubin. *Truth, Lies, and Public Health: How We Are Affected When Science and Politics Collide*. Westport, Conn.: Praeger, 2007.

Foucault, Michel. *Psychiatric Power: Lectures at the Collège de France, 1973–74*. Edited by Jacques Lagrange. Translated by Graham Burchell. New York: Picador, 2008.

———. *The History of Sexuality, Vol. 1: An Introduction*. New York: Vintage, 1990.

Franks, Angela. *Margaret Sanger's Eugenic Legacy: The Control of Female Fertility*. Jefferson, N.C.: McFarland, 2005.

Gaines, Ernest. *A Lesson Before Dying*. New York: Vintage, 2007.

Garrow, David J. *Liberty and Sexuality: The Right to Privacy and the Making of Roe v. Wade*. Berkeley: University of California Press, 1998.

Gates, Henry Louis, Jr. "The Passing of Anatole Broyard." Reprinted in Henry Louis Gates, Jr., *Thirteen Ways of Looking at a Black Man*, 180–214. New York: Random House, 1997.

Gherovici, Patricia. *The Puerto Rican Syndrome*. New York: Other Press, 2003.

Gibson, Lydialyle. "Long Way Home." *University of Chicago Magazine*, January–February 2008 (http://magazine.uchicago.edu).

Glantz, Leonard H. "Nontherapeutic Research with Children: Grimes v. Kennedy Krieger Institute." *American Journal of Public Health* 92, no. 7 (July 2002): 1070–73.

Gold, Michael. *A Conspiracy of Cells: One Woman's Immortal Legacy and the Medical Scandal It Caused*. Albany: State University of New York Press, 1986.

Goodman, Jordan, Anthony McElligott, and Lara Marks. "Making Bodies Useful: Historicizing Medical Experiments in the Twentieth Century." In their *Useful Bodies: Humans in the Service of Medical Science in the Twentieth Century*, Baltimore: Johns Hopkins University Press, 2003.

Gordon, Linda. *The Moral Property of Women: A History of Birth Control Politics in America*. Urbana: University of Illinois Press, 2002.

Gordon-Reed, Annette. *The Hemingses of Monticello: An American Family*. New York: Norton, 2008.

———. *Thomas Jefferson and Sally Hemings: An American Controversy*. Charlottesville: University of Virginia Press, 1997.

Haller, Mark. *Eugenics: Hereditarian Attitudes in American Thought*. New Brunswick, N.J.: Rutgers University Press, 1983.

Hampson, Lindsay A., and Ezekiel J. Emmanuel. "The Prognosis for Changes in End-of-Life Care after the Schiavo Case." *Health Affairs* 24, no. 4 (July 2005): 972–75.

Harris, Cheryl. "Whiteness as Property." *Harvard Law Review* 106, no. 8 (1993): 1709–95.

Harris, Trudier. "This Disease Called Strength." *Literature and Medicine* 14 (1995): 109–26.

Helly, Dorothy, and Susan Reverby, eds. *Gendered Domains: Beyond the Public and Private in Women's History*. Ithaca, N.Y.: Cornell University Press, 1992.

Henkin, Louis. "Privacy and Autonomy." *Columbia Law Review* 74 (1974): 1410–33.

Hill-Collins, Patricia. *Black Feminist Thought: Knowledge, Consciousness, and the Politics of Empowerment*. New York: Routledge, 2000.

Holloway, Karla FC. "Accidental Communities: Race, Ethics, and the Problem of PolyHeme. *American Journal of Bioethics* 6, no. 3 (2006): 7–17.

———. Codes of Conduct: *Race, Ethics, and the Color of Our Character*. New Brunswick, N.J.: Rutgers University Press, 1995.

———. "Nothing's Secret." *Duke Magazine*, May–June 2009: 45–46.

———. *Passed On: African American Mourning Stories; A Memorial*. Durham: Duke University Press, 2002.

———. "Private Bodies/Public Texts: Literature, Science, and States of Surveillance." *Literature and Medicine* 26, no. 1 (spring 2007): 269–76.

Hornblum, Allen. *Acres of Skin: Human Experiments at Holmesburg Prison*. New York: Routledge, 1998.

Horne, Jed. *Breach of Faith: Hurricane Katrina and the Near Death of a Great American City*. New York: Random House, 2006.

Huxley, Aldous. *Brave New World*. 1932. New York: Harper Perennial, 2006.

Ifill, Sherrilyn. *On the Courthouse Lawn: Confronting the Legacy of Lynching in the Twenty-first Century*. Boston: Beacon, 2008.

Inness, Julie C. *Privacy, Intimacy and Isolation*. New York: Oxford University Press, 1992.

Ishiguro, Kazuo. *Never Let Me Go*. New York: Vintage, 2005.

Jameson, Fredric. *The Political Unconscious: Narrative as Socially Symbolic Act*. Ithaca, N.Y.: Cornell University Press, 1982.

Jenkins, Candice. *Private Lives, Proper Relations: Regulating Black Intimacy*. Minneapolis: University of Minnesota Press, 2007.

Joh, Elizabeth. "Reclaiming 'Abandoned' DNA: The Fourth Amendment and Genetic Privacy." *Northwestern University Law Review* 100 (2006): 857–84.

Johnson, John. *Griswold v. Connecticut: Birth Control and the Constitutional Right to Privacy*. Lawrence: University Press of Kansas, 2005.

Jones, James H. *Bad Blood: The Tuskegee Syphilis Experiment*. New York: Free Press, 1993.

Junod, Suzanne, and Lara Marks. "Women's Trials: The Approval of the First Oral Contraceptive Pill in the United States and Great Britain." *Journal of the History of Medicine and Allied Sciences* 57, no. 2 (2002): 117–60.

Kahn, Jonathan. "Privacy as a Legal Principle of Identity Maintenance." *Seton Hall Law Review* 33 (2002–3): 371–410.

———. "Race in a Bottle." *Scientific American*, July 15, 2007: 40–45.

Kass, Nancy. "Public Health Ethics: From Foundations and Frameworks to Justice and Global Public Health." *Journal of Law, Medicine and Ethics* 32, no. 2 (2004): 232–42.

Katz, Jay, comp. *Experimentation with Human Beings: The Authority of the Investigator, Subject, Professions, and State in the Human Experimentation Process*. New York: Russell Sage Foundation, 1972.

Kipnis, Ken, Nancy King, and Robert Nelson. "An Open Letter to IRBs Considering Northfield Laboratories' PolyHeme Trial." *American Journal of Bioethics* 6, no. 3 (2006): 18–21.

Kittles, Rick, A. B. Baffoe-Bonnie, T. Y. Moses, C. M. Robbins, C. Ahaghotu, P. Huusko, C. Pettaway, S. Vijayakumar, J. Bennett, G. Hoke et al. "A Common Nonsense Mutation in *EphB2* Is Associated with Prostate Cancer Risk in African American Men with a Positive Family History." *Journal of Medical Genetics* 43, no. 6 (2006): 507–11.

Kittles, Rick, and Charmaine Royal. "The Genetics of African Americans: Implications for Disease Gene Mapping and Identity." In *Genetic Nature/Culture: Anthropology and Science beyond the Two-Culture Divide*, edited by Alan H. Goodman, Deborah Heath, and M. Susan Lindee, 219–33. Berkeley: University of California Press, 2003.

Kluchin, Rebecca. *Fit to Be Tied: Sterilization and Reproductive Rights in America 1950–1980*. New Brunswick: N.J.: Rutgers University Press, 2009.

Koerner, Brendan. "Blood Feud." *Wired*, September 2005. Wired.com.

Landecker, Hannah. *Culturing Life: How Cells Become Technologies*. Cambridge: Harvard University Press, 2007.

Lewis, Earl, and Heidi Aridizzone. *Love on Trial: An American Scandal in Black and White*. New York: Norton, 2001.

Liebler, Raizel. "Are You My Parent? Are You My Child? The Role of Genetics and Race in Defining Relationships after Reproductive Technological Mistakes." *DePaul Journal of Health Care Law* 5, no. 15 (2002): 42–52.

Lugosi, Charles. "Natural Disasters, Unnatural Deaths: The Killings on the Life-Care Floor at Tenet after Hurricane Katrina." *Issues in Law & Medicine* 23, no. 1 (2007): 71–85.

MacKinnon, Catherine. *Toward a Feminist Theory of the State*. Cambridge: Harvard University Press, 1991.

Marks, Lara. *Sexual Chemistry: A History of the Contraceptive Pill*. New Haven: Yale University Press, 2001.

———. "A 'Cage' of Ovulating Females": The History of the Early Oral Contraceptive Pill Clinical Trials, 1950–1959." In *Molecularizing Biology and Medicine: New Practices and Alliances, 1910s–1970s*, ed. Soraya De Chadarevian and Harmke Kamminga, 221–48. Amsterdam: Harwood Academic Press, 1998.

Mason, Alpheus. *Brandeis: A Free Man's Life*. New York: Viking, 1946.

Mason, J. K., and R. A. McCall Smith. *Law and Medical Ethics*. 2nd ed. London: Butterworth, 1987.

Mastroianni, Anna, and Jeffrey Kahn. "Risk and Responsibility: Ethics, Grimes v. Kennedy Krieger, and Public Health Research Involving Children. *American Journal of Public Health* 92, no. 7 (July 2002): 1073–76.

———. "Swinging on the Pendulum: Shifting Views of Justice in Human Subjects Research." *Hastings Center Report* 31, no. 3 (2001): 21–28.

May, Elaine Tyler. *Barren in the Promised Land*. Cambridge: Harvard University Press, 2007.

McDougall, Jennifer Fecio, and Martha Gorman. *Euthanasia: A Reference Handbook*. Contemporary World Issues. Santa Barbara, Calif.: ABC Clio, 2007.

McGregor, Deborah. *From Midwives to Medicine*. New Brunswick, N.J.: Rutgers University Press, 1998.

Mele, Christopher. *Civil Penalties, Social Consequences*. New York: Routledge, 2005.

Michie, Helena, and Naomi Cahn. *Confinements: Fertility and Infertility in Contemporary Culture*. New Brunswick, N.J.: Rutgers University Press, 1997.

Miles, Steven, and Allison August. "Courts, Gender and the Right to Die." *Law, Medicine & Health Care* 18 (spring/summer 1990): 85–95.

Morrison, Toni. *Jazz*. New York: Knopf, 1992.

———. "Unspeakable Things Unspoken: The Afro-American Presence in American Literature." *Michigan Quarterly Review* 28, no. 1 (1989): 1–35.

Moskowitz, Ellen, Bruce Jennings, and Daniel Callahan. "Long-Acting Contraceptives: Ethical Guidance for Policymakers and Health Care Providers." *Hastings Center Report* 25, no. 1 (January–February 1995): S1–8.

Nelson, Alondra. "BioScience, Genetic Genealogy Testing and the Pursuit of African Ancestry." In *Social Studies of Science* 38, no. 5 (2008): 759–83.

Nelson, Hilde Lindemann, ed. *Stories and Their Limits: Narrative Approaches to Bioethics*. New York: Routledge, 1997.

Nelson, Jennifer. *Women of Color and the Reproductive Rights Movement*. New York: New York University Press, 2003.

Nuland, Sherwin. *How We Die: Reflections on Life's Final Chapter*. New York: Vintage, 1995.

Nussbaum, Martha C. *Love's Knowledge: Essays on Philosophy and Literature*. New York: Oxford University Press, 1990.

Onwuachi-Willig, Angela. "A Beautiful Lie: Exploring *Rhinelander v. Rhinelander* as a Formative Lesson on Race, Identity, Marriage, and Family." *California Law Review* 95 (2007): 2393–458.

Paul, Diane B. *The Politics of Heredity: Essays on Eugenics, Biomedicine and the Nature-Nurture Debate*. Albany: State University of New York, 1998.

Pernick, Martin S. *A Calculus of Suffering: Pain, Professionalism, and Anesthesia in Nineteenth-century America*. New York: Columbia University Press, 1985.

Picoult, Jodi. *My Sister's Keeper*. New York: Washington Square Press, 2004.

Pine, Daniel S., G. A. Wasserman, J. Coplan, J. A. Fried, Y. Y. Huang, S. Kassir, L. Greenhill, D. Shaffer, and B. Parsons. "Platelet Serotonin 2A (5-HT2A) Receptor Characteristics and Parenting Factors for Boys at Risk for Delinquency: A Preliminary Report." *American Journal of Psychiatry* 153 (1996): 538–44.

Powers, Madison, and Ruth Faden. *Social Justice: The Moral Foundations of Public Health and Health Policy*. Oxford: Oxford University Press, 2006.

Quinlan, Julia Duane. *My Joy, My Sorrow: Karen Ann's Mother Remembers*. Cincinnati, Ohio: St. Anthony Messenger, 2006.

Racine, Eric, Rakesh Amaram, Matthew Seidler, Marta Karczewska, and Judy Illes. "Media Coverage of the Persistent Vegetative State and End-of-life Decision-making." *Neurology* 71 (2008): 1027–32.

Rao, Radhika. "Genes and Spleens: Property, Contract, or Privacy Rights in the Human Body?" *Journal of Law, Medicine and Ethics* 35, no. 3 (fall 2007): 371–82.

Reardon, Jenny. *Race to the Finish: Identity and Governance in an Age of Genomics*. Princeton: Princeton University Press, 2005.

Reverby, Susan M. *Examining Tuskegee: The Infamous Syphilis Study and Its Legacy*. Chapel Hill: University of North Carolina Press, 2009.

————, ed. *Tuskegee's Truths: Rethinking the Tuskegee Syphilis Study*. Chapel Hill: University of North Carolina Press, 2000.

Rise, Eric. *The Martinsville Seven: Race, Rape, and Capital Punishment*. Charlottesville: University of Virginia Press, 1998.

Roberts, Dorothy. *Killing the Black Body*. New York: Vintage, 1998.

————. "Punishing Drug Addicts Who Have Babies: Women of Color, Equality, and the Right of Privacy." *Harvard Law Review* 104, no. 7 (1991): 1419–82.

————. "Reconstructing the Patient: Starting with Women of Color." In *Feminism and Bioethics: Beyond Reproduction*, edited by Susan M. Wolf, 116–43. New York: Oxford University Press, 1996.

Rosser, Sue V. *Women's Health: Missing from U.S. Medicine*. Bloomington: Indiana University Press, 1994.

Rothman, David. *Strangers at the Bedside*. New York: Basic, 1992.

Royal, Charmaine. "'Race' and Ethnicity in Science, Medicine and Society." *Biosocieties* 1, no. 3 (2006): 325–28.

Rubenfeld, Jed. "The Right of Privacy." *Harvard Law Review* 102, no. 4 (February 1989): 737–807.

Sartin, Jeffrey. "J. Marion Sims: The Father of Gynecology: Hero or Villain?" *Southern Medical Journal* 97, no. 5 (2004): 500–5.

Satcher, David. "Our Commitment to Eliminate Racial and Ethnic Health Disparities." *Yale Journal of Health Policy, Law, and Ethics* 1, no. 1 (2001): 1–14.

Schneider, Elizabeth M. "The Violence of Privacy." *Connecticut Law Review* 23 (1991): 973–1001.

Schwartz, Marie. *Birthing a Slave: Motherhood and Medicine in the Antebellum South*. Cambridge: Harvard University Press, 2006.

Seaman, Barbara. *The Greatest Experiment Ever Performed on Women: Exploding the Estrogen Myth*. New York: Hyperion, 2003.

Shamir, Milette. *Inexpressible Privacy: The Interior Life of Antebellum American Literature*. Philadelphia: University of Pennsylvania Press, 2006.

Sims, J. Marion. *The Story of My Life*. New York: Appleton, 1884.

Skloot, Rebecca. "Henrietta's Dance." *Johns Hopkins Magazine*, April 2000 (http://magazine.jhu.edu/).

————. *The Immortal Life of Henrietta Lacks*. New York: Crown, 2010.

Smedley, Brian D., Adrienne Y. Stith, and Alan R. Nelson, eds. *Unequal Treatment: Confronting Racial and Ethnic Disparities in Health Care*. Washington: National Academy Press, 2003.

Smith-Pryor, Elizabeth. *Property Rites: The Rhinelander Trial, Passing, and the Protection of Whiteness*. Chapel Hill: University of North Carolina Press, 2009.

"Sterilized: Why?" *Time*, July 23, 1973.

Tallbear, Kimberly. "Narratives of Race and Indigeneity in the Genographic Project." *Journal of Law, Medicine and Ethics* 35, no. 3 (fall 2007): 412–24.

Vaughn, Paul. *The Pill on Trial.* New York: Coward-McCann, 1970.

Vince, Gaia. "White IVF Couple Have Black Twins." *New Scientist,* July 8, 2002 (http://www.newscientist.com).

Wailoo, Keith, and Stephen Pemberton. *The Troubled Dream of Genetic Medicine.* Baltimore: Johns Hopkins University Press, 2006.

Wald, Priscilla. *Contagious: Cultures, Carriers, and the Outbreak Narrative.* Durham: Duke University Press, 2008.

Wall, Lewis. "The Medical Ethics of Dr. J. Marion Sims." *Journal of Medical Ethics* 32 (2006): 346–50.

Warren, Samuel, and Louis Brandeis. "The Right to Privacy." *Harvard Law Review* 4, no. 5 (December 15, 1890): 193–220.

Washington, Harriet. *Medical Apartheid: The Dark History of Medical Experimentation.* New York: Random House, 2007.

Weindling, Paul. *Nazi Medicine and the Nuremberg Trials: From Medical War Crimes to Informed Consent.* New York: Palgrave Macmillan, 2006.

White House. "President Clinton Announces the Completion of the First Survey of the Entire Human Genome." Press release, Office of the Press Secretary. June 25, 2000.

Whitman, Walt. *Song of Myself and Other Poems.* 1855. Ed. Robert Hass. Berkeley, Calif.: Counterpoint, 2010.

Wiegman, Robyn. "Intimate Publics, Race, Property and Personhood." *American Literature* 74, no. 4 (December 2002): 859–85.

Woolf, Steven, Robert Johnson, George Fryer Jr., George Rust, and David P. Satcher. *American Journal of Public Health* 98 (September 2008), Supplement 1: S26–S28.

Wright, William. *Critical Reflections on Black History.* Westport, Conn.: Praeger, 2002.

Legal Cases

Bowers v. Hardwick, 478 U.S. 186 (1986)
California v. Greenwood, 486 U.S. 35 (1988)
Doe v. Kamehameha Schools/Bernice Pauahi Bishop, 416 F. 3d (2005)
Eisenstadt v. Baird, 405 U.S. 438 (1972)
Grimes v. Kennedy Krieger Institute, Inc. 782 A2d 807 (2001)
Griswold v. Connecticut, 381 U.S. 479 (1965)
Harnicher v. Utah Medical Center, 962 P.2d 67 (Utah) (1998)

Hyman v. Jewish Chronic Disease Hospital 15 N.Y. 2d 317, 206 N.E. 2d 338 (1965)

In Re Grand Jury Subpoena, Judith Miller, 397 F. 3d 964, 970 (D.C. Cir. 2005)

In re Quinlan, 348 A.2d 801, NJ: Superior Court (1975)

In re Quinlan 70 N.J. 10, 355 A.2d 647 (1976)

Lawrence v. Texas, 539 U.S. 558 (2003)

Moore v. Regents of the University of California (51 Cal. 3d 120; 271 Cal. Rptr. 146; 793 P.2d 479 (1990)

NC Dep't of Corr v. NC Med Board (51PAO8) May 1, 2009

Pavesich v. New England Life Insurance Co., 50 S.E. 68 (1905)

Perry-Rogers v. Fasano, 715 N.Y.S. 2d 19 (N.Y. App. Div., 2000)

Petitioner Affidavit at 1, *State of Louisiana v. Anna M. Pou, Lori L. Budo, and Cheri A. Landry* No. 471829 (July 17, 2006)

Planned Parenthood of Southeastern Pennsylvania v. Casey, 505 U.S. 833 (1992)

Plessy v. Ferguson, 163 U.S. 537 (1896)

Relf v. Weinberger, 565 F.2d 722 (1977)

Rhinelander v. Rhinelander, 219 NYS 548, 219 AD 189, 219 App. Div. 189 (1927)

Roberson v. Rochester Folding Box Co. 64 N.E. 442 (N.Y. 1902)

Roe v. Wade, 410 U.S. 113 (1973)

Tucker v. Blease, 97 S.C. 303 (1913)/*Buck v. Bell* 274 US 200 (1927)

US v. Kincade, 379 F. 3d 813—Court of Appeals, 9th Circuit (2004)

Index

racial marriage, 44; *A Lesson before Dying* (Gaines), 141–43; motherhood and, 57–59, 62–63; neutrality of, 19–20; in popular media, 10; reproduction and, 31, 35, 47, 61, 64–65, 114, 121; right to die and, 1–2, 155–56. *See also* privacy, right to

law of the body, 8

Lawrence v. Texas, 15

lead abatement research, 133–35

Lesson before Dying, A (Gaines), 140–43

Levesque, William, 18–19

Lewis, Meriwether, 68

liberty, right to, 28

LifeCare, 157–61, 167–71

literature, fictional. *See* fiction, literary

Lord of the Rings (Tolkien), 182n10

Lowenstein Center for the Study and Prevention of Childhood Disruptive Behavior Disorders, 119

MacKinnon, Catherine, 177n12

mapping: the body, *Wit* (Edson), 152–53; death, "Summer Tragedy" (Bontemps), 166; the human genome, 68–70, 71, 76–78; human migratory patterns, 81, 92–93

marriage: contraceptive rights and, 62; interracial, 39–42, 44–45, 64; privacy rights accorded to, 61. *See also* domestic privacy

Mason, J. K., 62

Massachusetts General Hospital, 129

Mastroianni, Anna, 111–12, 115, 123

May, Elaine, 55

McCormick, Katherine, 49

McGregor, Deborah, 176n3

McManus, Angela, 160–61, 164

measles vaccine research (NIH), 125–27

Medical Apartheid (Washington), xvi–xvii

medical care: race and poverty and, 115, 156–64, 167–71; racialization of, 32, 113, 125, 187n73, 189n31

medical ethics: confidentiality issues in, 125; emotions role in, 110–11; HeLa cell line and, 2–6, 19; Helsinki declarations effect on, 125; narrative as vehicle for analysis in, 107–10; in nineteenth century, 31–32; for physicians and executions, 140; race factor in, 123–27; research guidelines for, 103, 105, 147; standards of care in emergency situations, 168–70; vulnerable populations and principled application of, 49–52, 82, 103–6, 156–64. *See also* informed consent

medical experiment, 102–3

medical experimentation. *See* black men; children, medical experimentation on; clinical trials; women's bodies

medical research: ethical guidelines, 103, 105, 147; gender variable in, 83; incentives and, 113, 119–20, 135; language of, 101–2; race-based, 83, 89–90, 95–97, 129–32

medicine: fiction as illustration of, 10–14; individualized, 76, 78, 95–97; neutrality in, 6–7; in popular media, 3, 10; social order and practices of, 59. *See also* patients; public health

Karla FC Holloway is James B. Duke
Professor of English and professor of law,
African & African American studies, and
women's studies at Duke University.

Library of Congress
Cataloging-in-Publication Data
Holloway, Karla F. C.
Private bodies, public texts : race, gender, and
a cultural bioethics / Karla FC Holloway.
p. cm.
Includes bibliographical references and index.
ISBN 978-0-8223-4894-8 (cloth : alk. paper)—
ISBN 978-0-8223-4917-4 (pbk. : alk. paper)
1. African Americans—Medical care—Moral
and ethical aspects. 2. Medical ethics—United
States. 3. Social status—Health aspects—
United States. 4. Health and race. I. Title.
RA448.5.N4H655 2011
174.20973—dc22
2010031784